46 Deliciou Juice Recipes

A Complete Recipe Book of Healthy, Tasty Juice Ideas!

Table of Contents

Introduction 5

1 – Ginger and Apple Detox Juice 7
2 – Apple and Spinach Detox Juice 9
3 – Easy Start Carrot Detox Juice 11
4 – Carrot and Beet Detox Juice 13
5 – Creamsicle® Orange Detox Juice 15
6 – Kale and Lemon Detox Juice 17
7 – Allergy Fighter Detox Juice 19
8 – Alkaline Apple and Broccoli Boost Juice 21
9 – Lemonade and Spinach Detox Juice 23
10 – Sweet Beet and Lemon Detox Juice 25
11 – Red Zinger Apple Carrot Detox Juice 27
12 – Carrot and Kiwi Detox Cleanse Juice 29
13 – Kid-Approved Apple and Orange Detox Juice 31
14 – New Start Apple and Kale Detox Juice 33
15 – Zesty Lemon and Apple Detox Juice 35
16 – Summer Pineapple and Ginger Detox Juice 37
17 – Pineapple and Carrot Detox Juice 39
18 – Super Cucumber and Lime Detox Juice 41
19 – Ultimate Green Detox Juice 43
20 – Apple Cucumber Detox Juice 45
21 – Turmeric and Carrot Detox Juice 47

22 – Anti-Inflammatory Detox Juice Blend 49

23 – Orange and Ginger Detox Juice 51

24 – Pear and Kale Detox Juice 53

25 – Sweet Apple and Carrot Detox Juice 55

26 – Healthy Beet Detox Juice 57

27 – Orange-Pineapple-Carrot Detox Juice 59

28 – Zingy Ginger Detox Juice 61

29 – Almond Strawberry Detox Juice 63

30 – Tropical Mint Detox Juice 65

31 – Fruit-Free Detox Juice 67

32 – Super Natural Detox Juice 69

33 – Healthy Green Detox Juice 71

34 – Cucumber Carrot Detox Juice 73

35 – Great Greens Detox Juice 75

36 – Cabbage Carrot Detox Juice 77

37 – Tropical Pineapple Detox Juice 79

38 – Healthy Skin Detox Juice 81

39 – Energy Boost Detox Juice 83

40 – Full Body Health Detox Juice 85

41 – Chia Berry Detox Juice 87

42 – Liver Cleanse Detox Juice 89

43 – Earthy Taste Detox Juice 91

44 – Sweet Veggie Detox Juice 93

45 – Healthy Ginger Lemon Juice 95
46 – Grapefruit and Spinach Detox Juice 97
Conclusion 99

Introduction

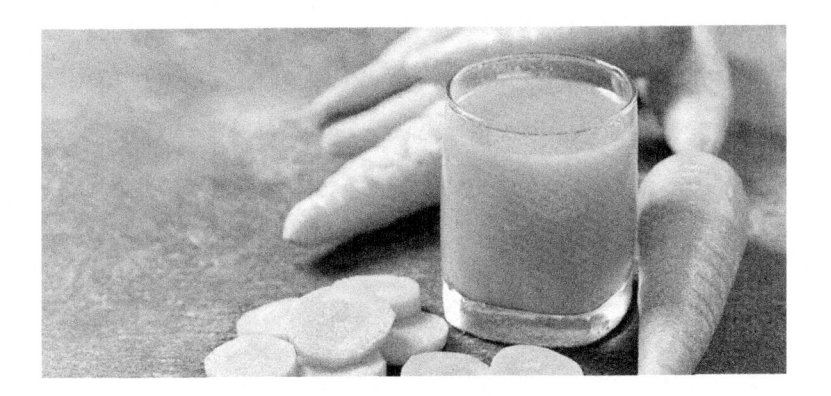

Why choose detox juice to maintain a healthy body?

Detox juice is SO nutritious, extracted from fresh vegetables and fruits. In this cookbook, we'll be focusing on using a juicer to more easily prepare detox juice.

If you're just starting out, experts recommend that you do a three-day cleanse, drinking only water and juice. This gives your digestive tract and liver the time they need to detoxify your body. During your cleanse, try to drink a glass every two to two and a half hours. Be consistent in your drinking. If you skip one, it could affect your body's blood sugar levels.

Detox juice is wonderful for losing weight, but it's also a valuable way to cleanse your body of the toxins it takes in from the environment we all live in and the foods you usually eat.

Most people don't reap the benefits of including healthy produce in their daily diet. Making and drinking detox juice is an easy way to get the daily servings of vegetables and fruits that your body thirsts for. Detox juice will provide the extra nutrition you need in your diet, and that may otherwise be lacking.

Detoxing through juicing is an easy way to get healthy and stay healthy, without cutting calories or counting points. It gives your body what it was designed to live on. Let's juice!

1 – Ginger and Apple Detox Juice

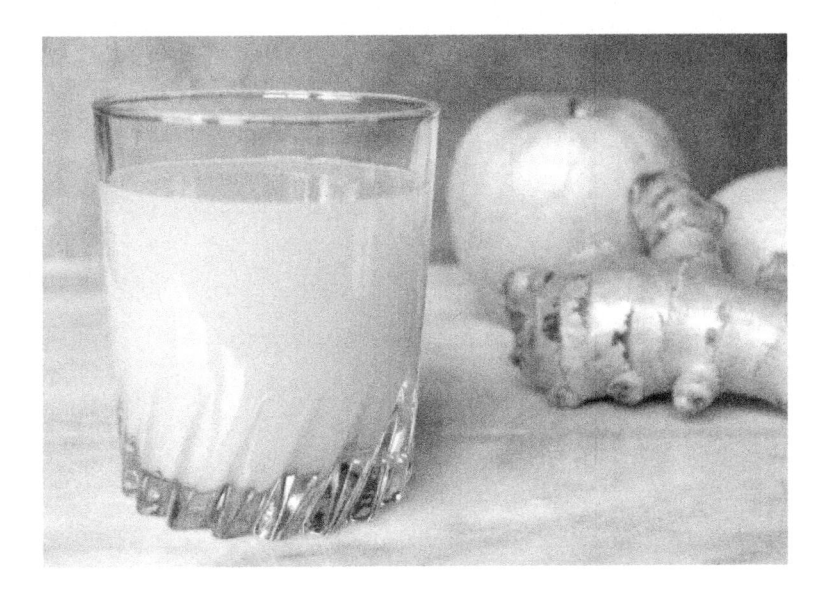

This is a recipe I go to often, particular if my stomach is giving me problems. It has amazing taste and the ingredients fill it with nutrients. Ginger is one of the most versatile spices. Just 1/2 inch or so can alleviate nausea from such causes as morning sickness and post-surgical nausea, as well as nausea from travel sickness or anxiety.

Makes 2 Servings

Prep Time: 10-12 minutes

Ingredients:

- 2 celery stalks
- 3 apples, medium
- 1 cucumber, medium
- 1 cup of spinach, baby
- 1 peeled lime
- 1 piece of 1-inch diameter ginger root

Instructions:

1. Wash veggies and fruits before you juice.

2. Cut the veggies and fruits into 2-inch pieces, so the juicer can work more effectively.

3. Place produce in machine. Turn it on and allow it to run till it has extracted all juice.

4. Enjoy when juicer is done or chill and drink later.

2 – Apple and Spinach Detox Juice

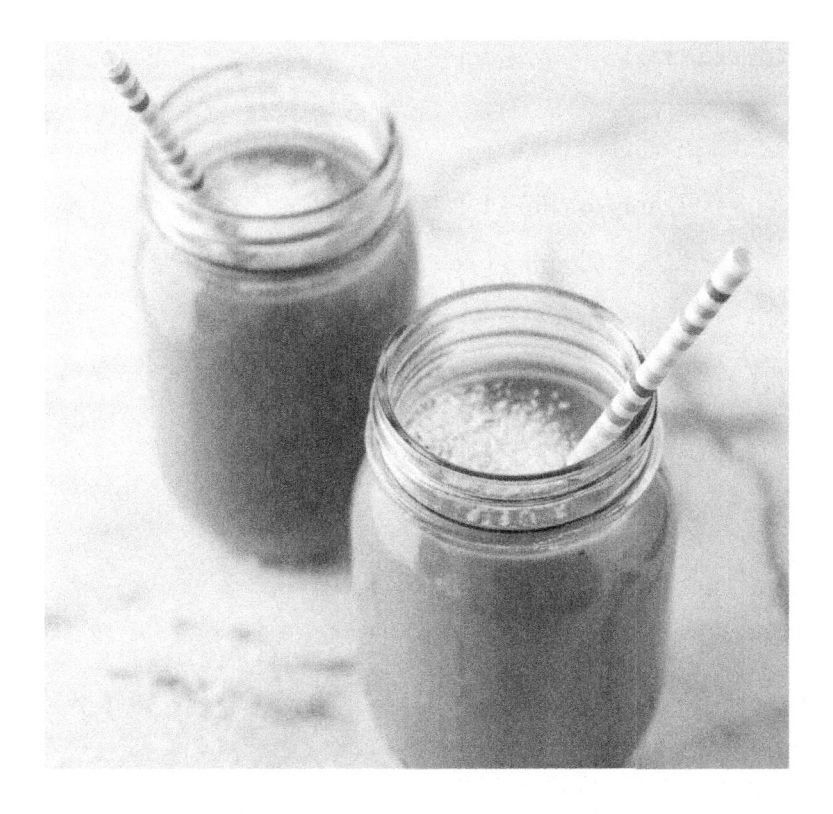

This recipe combines green apples and spinach for an alkalizing detox juice. The spinach has a mild taste and is full of nutrients. The ginger and lemon add some zing. The cucumbers contribute water rich in minerals, while the apple taste adds sweetness and tartness that balances the other flavors.

Makes 4 Servings

Prep Time: 10-12 minutes

Ingredients:

- 6 celery stalks
- 2 cups of spinach leaves, baby
- 1/2 of 1 lemon, peeled
- 2 cucumbers, large
- 1 to 2-inch ginger piece
- 2 apples, medium
- 1/4 to 1/2 cup of parsley, leaves only

Instructions:

1. Wash the produce.

2. Prep it and chop as needed.

3. Add ingredients to your juicer.

4. Serve cold.

3 – Easy Start Carrot Detox Juice

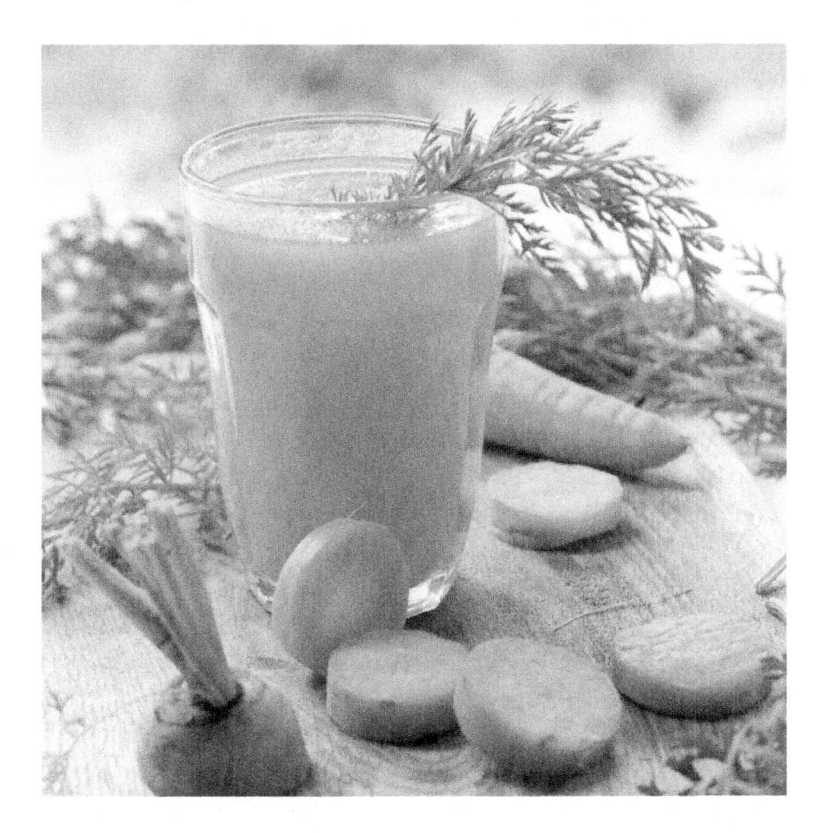

This is an excellent choice for those who are beginners to juicing. It has simple ingredients, plus the flavors are delicious and not overwhelming. Carrots have SO many benefits for your health. They aid in eye health and are linked to the lowering of cholesterol levels.

Makes 2 Servings

Prep Time: 7-10 minutes

Ingredients:

- 4 stalks of celery
- 3 carrots, medium
- 2 apples, medium

Instructions:

1. Wash produce to ensure it is clean.

2. Add to your juicer.

3. Process into detox juice.

4 – Carrot and Beet Detox Juice

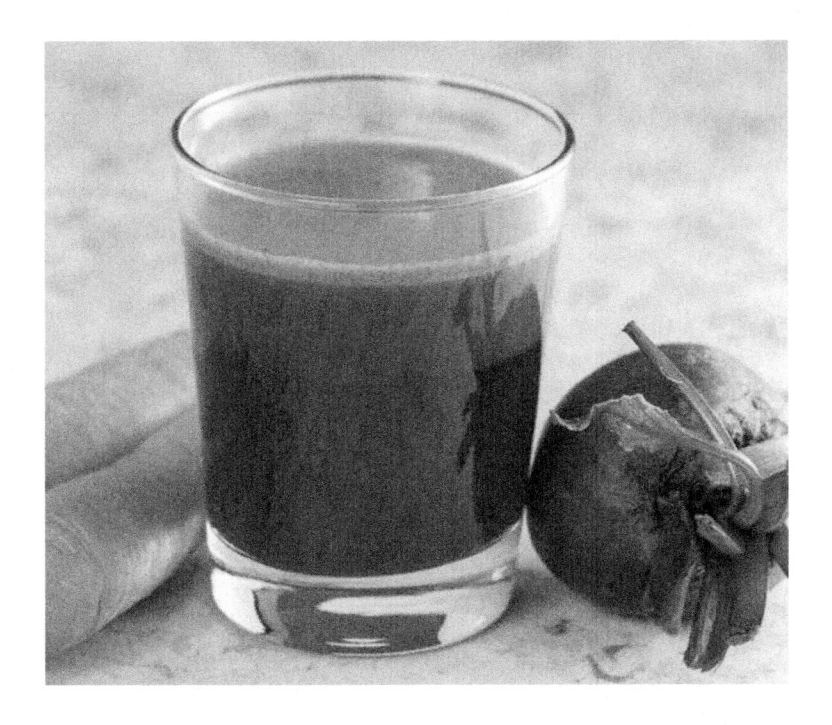

This juice has balanced flavor and it's a bit sweet from the sweet beets and apples, with ginger's signature kick. If you don't like ginger, you can use less or use none at all. You can always tweak the amounts of ingredients in recipes, to make detox juices you enjoy drinking.

Makes 4 Servings

Prep Time: 10-12 minutes

Ingredients:

- 6 carrots, medium
- 2 or 3 apples, medium to large
- 1/2 lemon, no peel
- 1 or 2 inches of ginger

Instructions:

1. Wash veggies and fruits before you juice.

2. Cut the veggies and fruits into 2-inch pieces, if you like, so the juicer can work more effectively.

3. Place produce in machine. Turn it on and allow it to run till it has extracted all juice.

4. Enjoy drinking when juicer is done or chill and drink later.

5 – Creamsicle® Orange Detox Juice

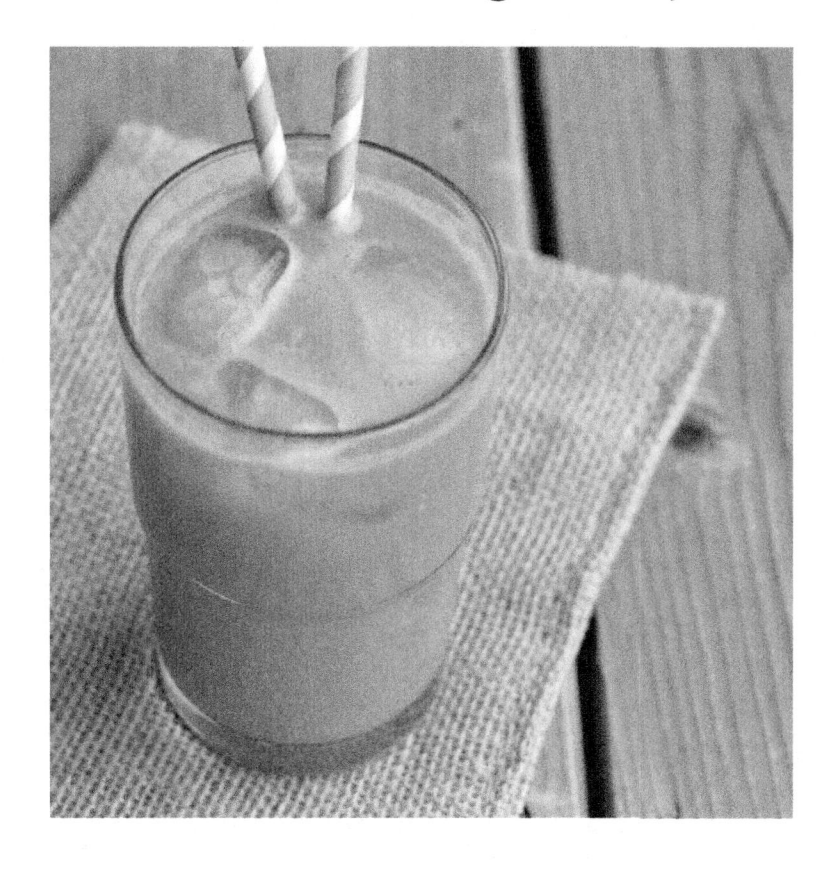

Remember Creamsicles®, those great orange ice cream bars? If you're old enough, you will. You can still find them in some stores today. This juice is every bit as delicious and creamy as the bars that give it the name. If you like, these can be frozen in popsicle molds, and you'll have a wonderful frozen treat to eat. For nutrient benefit, pears offer potassium, copper, vitamin C and vitamin K.

Makes 2 Servings

Prep Time: 7-10 minutes

Ingredients:

- 3 celery stalks
- 2 apples, medium
- 2 pears, medium
- 1 peeled orange
- 1 x 5-inch long sweet potato

Instructions:

1. Clean the produce and cut as needed.

2. Add ingredients to your juicer.

3. Process into healthy detox juice.

6 – Kale and Lemon Detox Juice

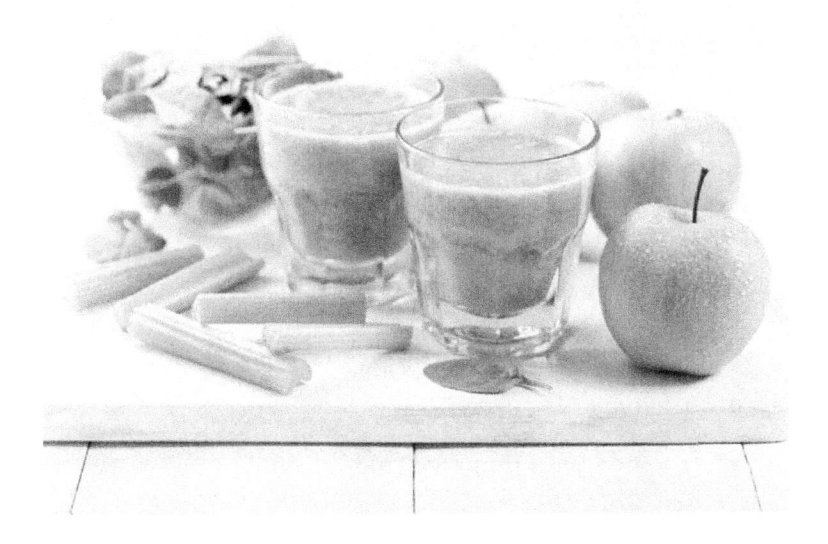

This tasty juice is packed with antioxidants, vitamins and minerals, and the kale gives your immunity a boost. Kale also contains chlorophyll, which is a natural blood cleanser. The apples are great for keeping the intestinal tract clear, while the lemon will clear toxins from your liver. To top it off, cucumber is hydrating and refreshing to drink.

Makes 1 Serving

Prep Time: 6-8 minutes

Ingredients:

- 1 handful of chopped spinach leaves
- 3 chopped leaves of kale, de-stemmed
- 1 bunch of chopped parsley
- 1 cup of romaine lettuce, chopped
- 2 chopped celery sticks
- 1/2 cucumber, English if available
- 1-inch piece of ginger, fresh
- 1 halved, de-seeded apple
- 1 lemon with removed rind

Instructions:

1. Wash the produce, then prep and chop as needed.

2. Add ingredients to your juicer.

3. Serve cold.

7 – Allergy Fighter Detox Juice

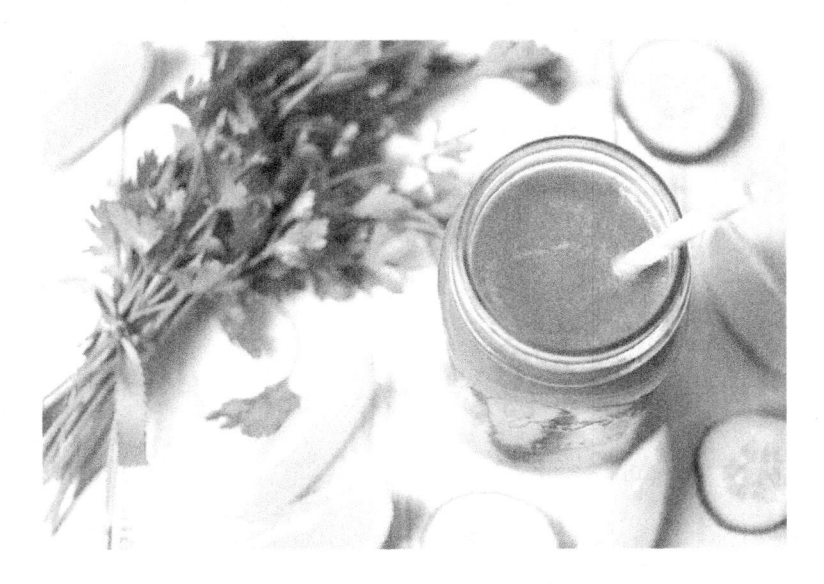

Do you have seasonal allergies? This detox juice till help you out. It boasts vitamin C, to help fight allergies, in the grapes, pineapples and lemon. Parsley is also an excellent source of iron, folate, vitamin A, vitamin C and vitamin K.

Makes 2 Servings

Prep Time: 10 minutes

Ingredients:

- 1 cup of pineapple
- 1 cucumber

- 1 cup of grapes, seedless
- 1 lemon
- 1 apple, medium
- 1/2 cup of parsley
- 1 sprig of mint, if desired

Instructions:

1. Clean your produce well.

2. Chop where needed.

3. Add ingredients to electric juicer.

4. Process the produce into detox juice.

8 – Alkaline Apple and Broccoli Boost Juice

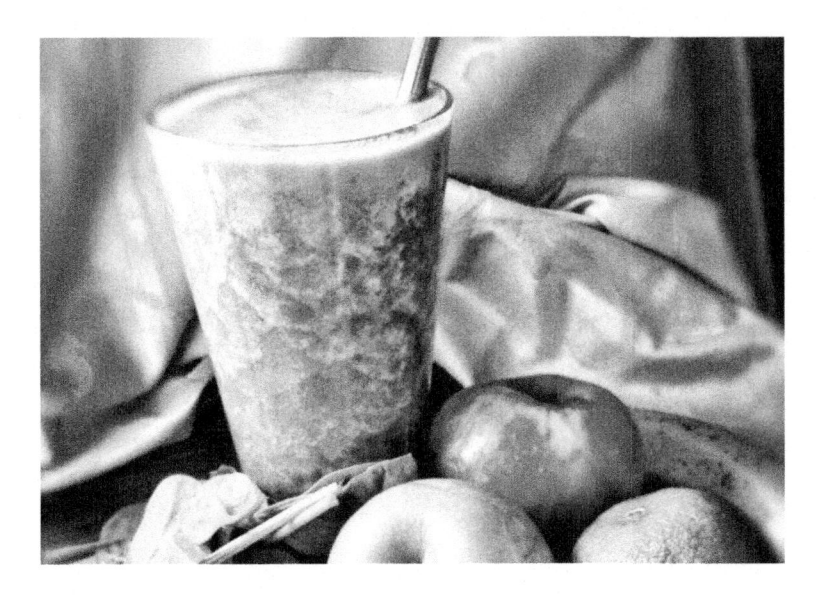

This is a sweet juice that works great for detoxing. It's high in iron, vitamin K and folate. The broccoli helps to oxygenate your blood and contains sufficient vitamin C to help your body absorb healthy iron. Broccoli leaves have vitamin A and vitamin C, which are super antioxidants.

Makes 2 Servings

Prep Time: 10 minutes

Ingredients:

- 2 celery stalks
- 1/2 cucumber
- 1 cup of broccoli florets
- 1 cup of lettuce, your fav type
- 1/2 lime, peeled
- 1 apple, green

Instructions:

1. Wash the vegetables and fruits well.

2. Place ingredients in your juicer.

3. Blend the juice well and chill if you like before serving.

9 – Lemonade and Spinach Detox Juice

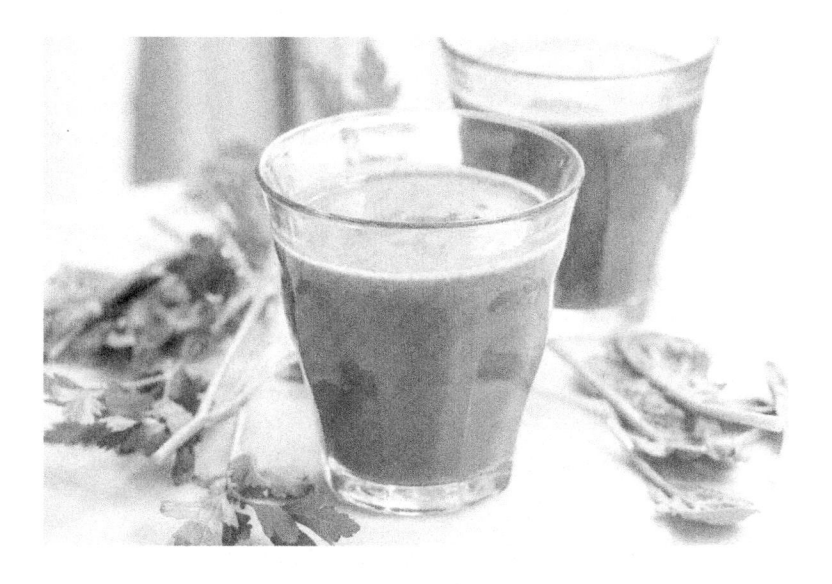

This is a popular detox juice that gives you lots of energy. It's healthy, too. If you prefer a sweeter taste, you can add a bit of honey. The kale leaves are low in calories and high in the number of nutrients offered. It's a very nutrient-dense food.

Makes 2 Servings

Prep Time: 8-10 minutes

Ingredients:

- 2 celery stalks
- 1 cup of spinach, baby
- 1 piece of ginger, fresh
- 4 kale leaves
- 1 lemon, rind removed
- 2 apples, quartered

Instructions:

1. Wash veggies and fruits before you juice.

2. Cut the veggies and fruits into 2-inch pieces, so the juicer can work more effectively.

3. Place produce in machine. Turn it on and allow it to run till it has extracted all juice.

4. Enjoy when juicer is done or chill and drink later.

10 – Sweet Beet and Lemon Detox Juice

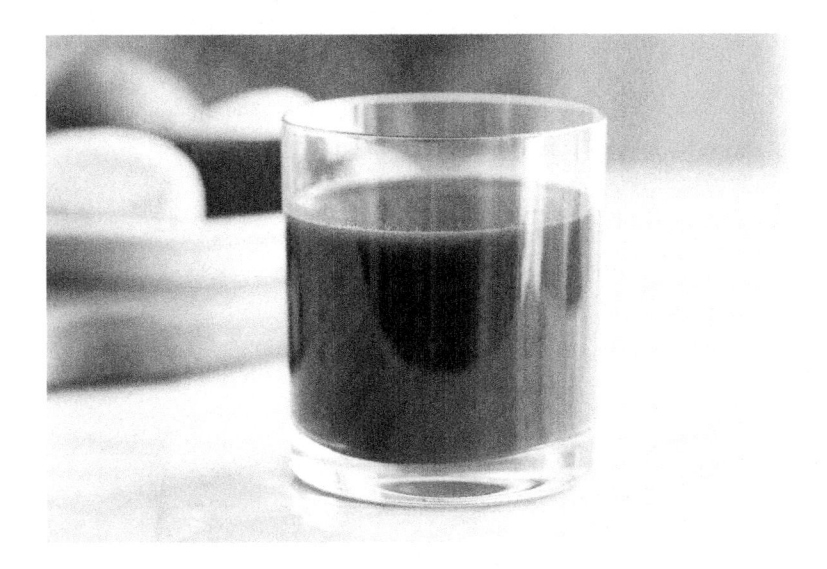

The beets in this detox juice are earthy and sweet, and the ginger offers its well-known zing. Beets have their own natural sweetness, so you don't need to add a lot of fruits to improve the taste.

Makes 2 Servings

Prep Time: 10 minutes

Ingredients:

- 2 carrots, medium
- 1 beet, red
- 1/2 lemon
- 3 celery stalks
- 1 apple, green
- 1/3-inch piece of ginger

Instructions:

1. Wash your produce well.

2. Place veggies and fruits into a juicer.

3. Blend till well juiced.

4. Chill before serving, if you like.

11 – Red Zinger Apple Carrot Detox Juice

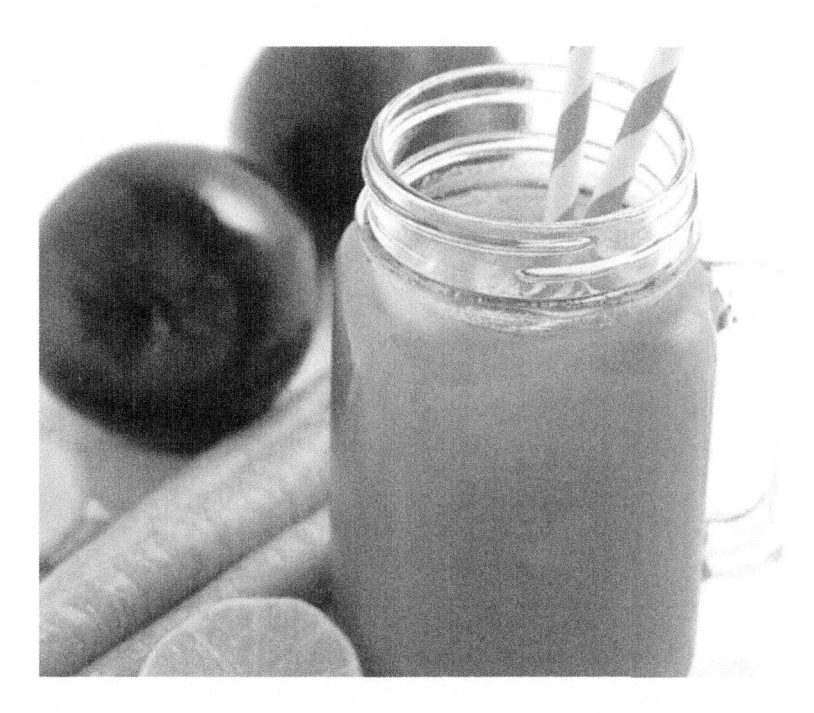

This is a wonderful juice to begin your days with. The fruits and vegetables offer excellent nutrition and provide the juice with natural good taste. The lemons give it a little kick. The beets, of course, are excellent sources of vitamin C, iron, manganese, potassium and folate.

Makes 2 Servings

Prep Time: 10 minutes

Ingredients:

- 2 carrots, medium
- 2 lemons, rind removed
- 2 beets
- 2 apples, green

Instructions:

1. Wash your vegetables and fruits so you're not drinking residual farm chemicals.

2. Cut produce into chunks, if you desire. Remove peels and rinds.

3. Place produce in juicer.

4. Process detox juice and serve chilled.

12 – Carrot and Kiwi Detox Cleanse Juice

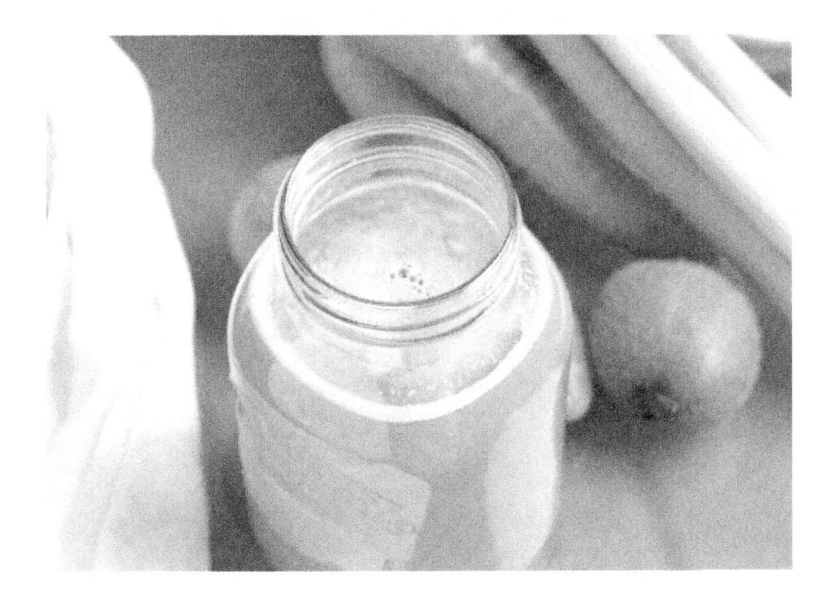

Carrots give your detox juice great taste, and they're also loaded with beneficial vitamins. They help you retain healthy eyes and skin, and they contain vitamin A, along with other nutrients that nourish your skin and body both.

Makes 2 Servings

Prep Time: 10 minutes

Ingredients:

- 1/3-inch ginger, fresh
- 4 carrots, medium
- 1/2 lemon
- 1 apple, green
- 2 celery stalks
- 1 kiwi
- 1/2 cup of sprouts
- 1/2 cucumber
- 1/2 cup of parsley leaves

Instructions:

1. Wash your ingredients thoroughly.

2. Place into juicer and blend together well.

3. Serve when ready or chilled.

13 – Kid-Approved Apple and Orange Detox Juice

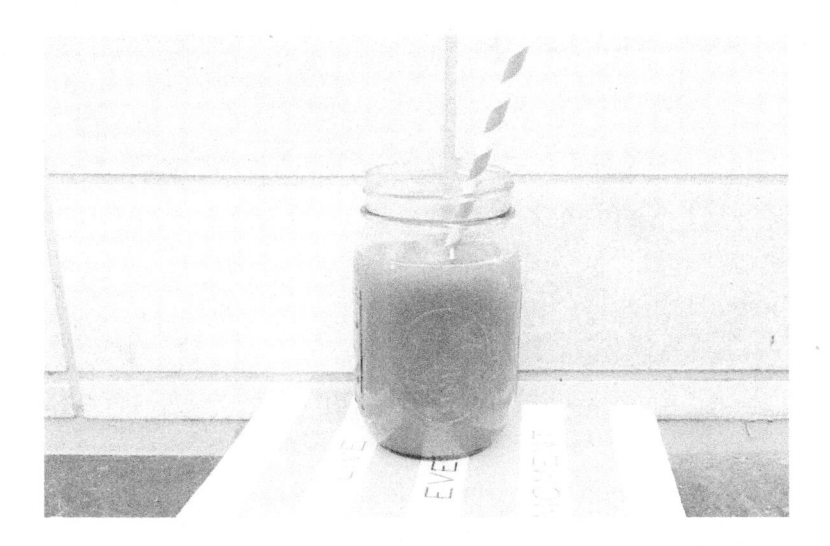

Kids will never drink detox juice, right? Wrong – kids (the ones I've served) love this recipe, since it's quite sweet. The fruits mask the veggie taste, making the overall taste palatable even for little ones. The spinach offers numerous vitamins and minerals. It also contains calcium, iron, folic acid, vitamin K, vitamin C and carotenoids.

Makes 2 Servings

Prep Time: 10 minutes

Ingredients:

- 1 peeled lemon
- 2 peeled oranges
- 1 quartered apple, green
- 1 kale leaf
- 1 cup of spinach, baby

Instructions:

1. Wash veggies and fruits before you juice.

2. Cut the veggies and fruits into 2-inch pieces, so the juicer can work more effectively.

3. Place produce in machine. Turn it on and allow it to run till it has extracted all juice.

4. Enjoy when juicer is done or chill and drink later.

14 – New Start Apple and Kale Detox Juice

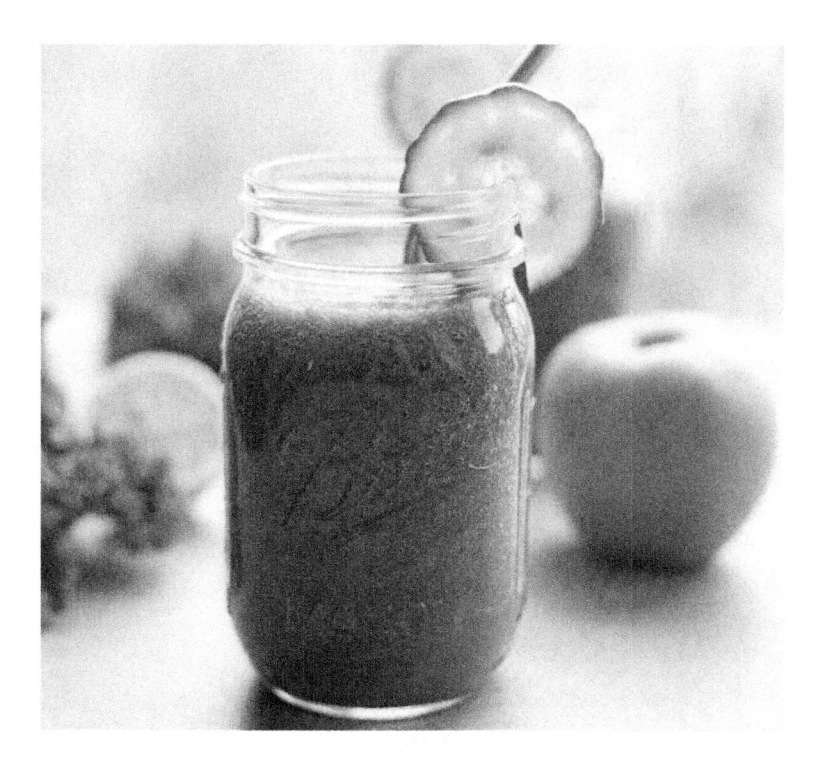

This apple and kale juice is easy and quick to make, and the ingredients are healthy for you. It's a great breakfast drink to start off your day. Many people don't appreciate bananas in their juices, and this one is banana free.

Makes 2 Servings

Prep Time: 10 minutes

Ingredients:

- 1/2 cucumber
- 2 celery stalks
- 1 cup of cilantro, fresh
- 1/2 lime, rind removed
- 1 apple, green
- 1 cup of kale

Instructions:

1. Wash ingredients thoroughly.

2. Place in juicer.

3. Blend together well.

4. Serve when done or chilled.

15 – Zesty Lemon and Apple Detox Juice

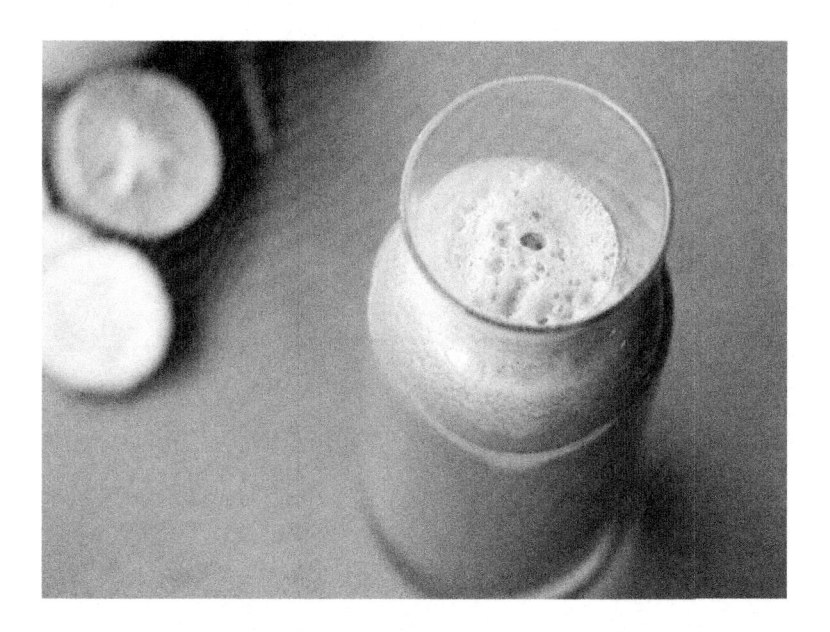

This tangy but light detox juice is surprisingly tasty, and another wonderful choice for your breakfast time juice. It contains antioxidants in lemons and apples and cucumbers offer vitamin K and other health benefits.

Makes 2 Servings

Prep Time: 7-10 minutes

Ingredients:

- 2 peeled, halved lemons, rind removed
- 4 quartered apples, green
- 2 halved cucumbers
- 1 cup of water, filtered

Instructions:

1. Wash off your fruits and vegetable.

2. Half or quarter cut as described in ingredients. Remove peels and rinds.

3. Place all the ingredients in your juicer.

4. Process into delicious detox juice.

5. Drink right away or chill first.

16 – Summer Pineapple and Ginger Detox Juice

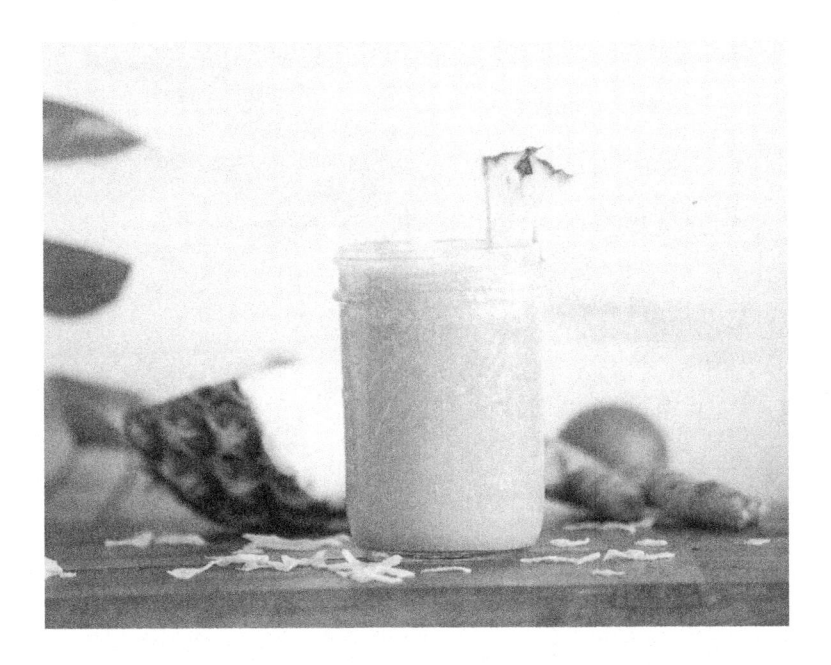

This ginger and pineapple juice is simply delicious. It's fresh, and still packed with many nutrients. Blending the ginger and pineapple together is easy to do in a blender, too, if you don't have a juicer.

Makes 2 Servings

Prep Time: 10 minutes

Ingredients:

- 1/2 lemon, rind removed
- 1 cup of pineapple, no rind, stem or core
- 2 celery stalks
- 2 carrots, medium
- 1/3 inch of ginger, fresh

Instructions:

1. Wash the vegetables and fruits well.

2. Slice or chop as needed.

3. Place ingredients in juicer and blend thoroughly.

4. Chill, then serve.

17 – Pineapple and Carrot Detox Juice

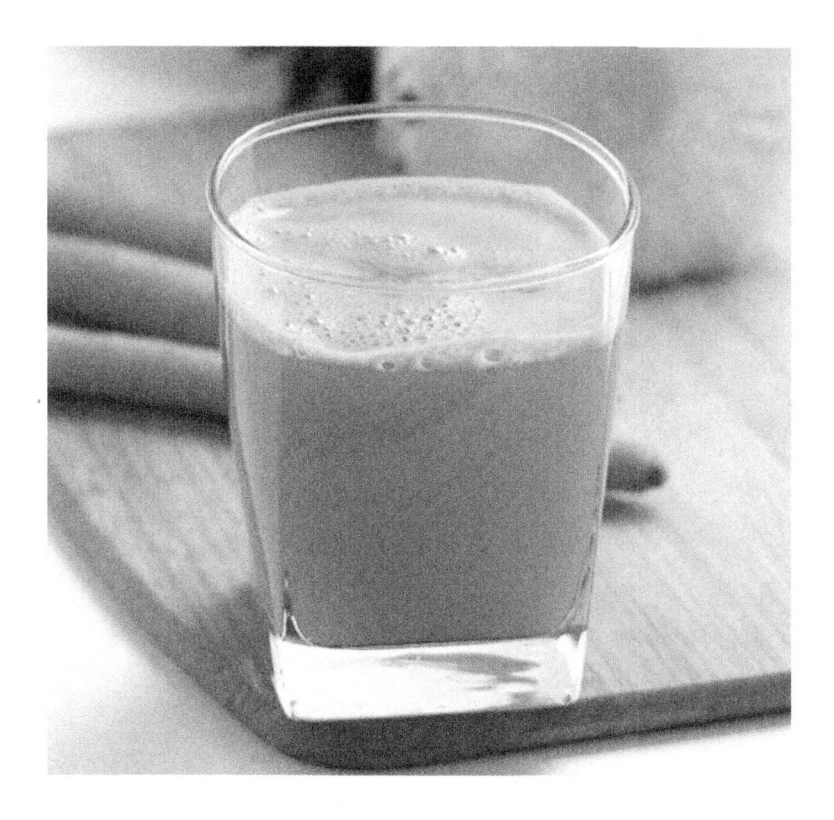

This is another detox juice that you can serve almost anyone, since it's delicious. It also is filled with nutrients like antioxidants, vitamins and minerals. Carrots are a major source for vitamin A, and they also have vitamin B and vitamin K, along with potassium. Carrot juice is actually sweet and it balances the apples' tartness.

Makes 2 Servings

Prep Time: 8-10 minutes

Ingredients:

- 1 quartered apple, large
- 1/4 can of chunked pineapple
- 2 fresh ginger pieces
- 2 carrots, large

Instructions:

1. Wash the fruits and vegetables well.

2. Chop or cut ingredients into chunks, if necessary for your juicer.

3. Remove peels and rinds.

4. Place all the ingredients into your juicer.

5. Process into detox juice.

18 – Super Cucumber and Lime Detox Juice

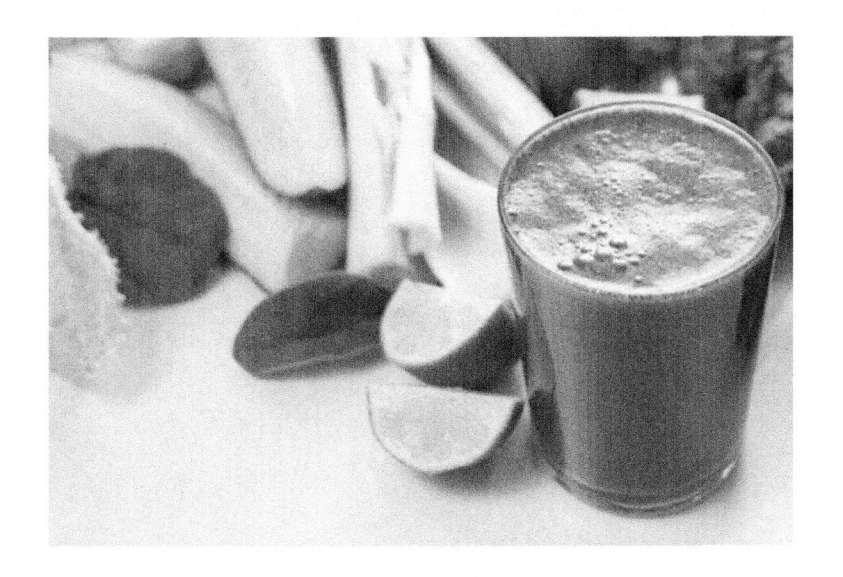

This is an easy, cooling detox juice, especially in the summer months. While some people prefer eating vegetables cooked, these juiced veggies and fruits are especially refreshing.

Makes 2 Servings

Prep Time: 10 minutes

Ingredients:

- 3/4 cucumber
- 2/3 inch of turmeric, fresh

- 1 apple, green
- 1/2 lime, no rind
- 1 cup of spinach, baby
- 2 beets, golden

Instructions:

1. Wash veggies and fruits before you juice.

2. Cut the veggies and fruits into 2-inch pieces, so the juicer can work more effectively.

3. Place produce in machine. Turn it on and allow it to run till it has extracted all juice.

4. Enjoy when juicer is done or chill and drink later.

19 – Ultimate Green Detox Juice

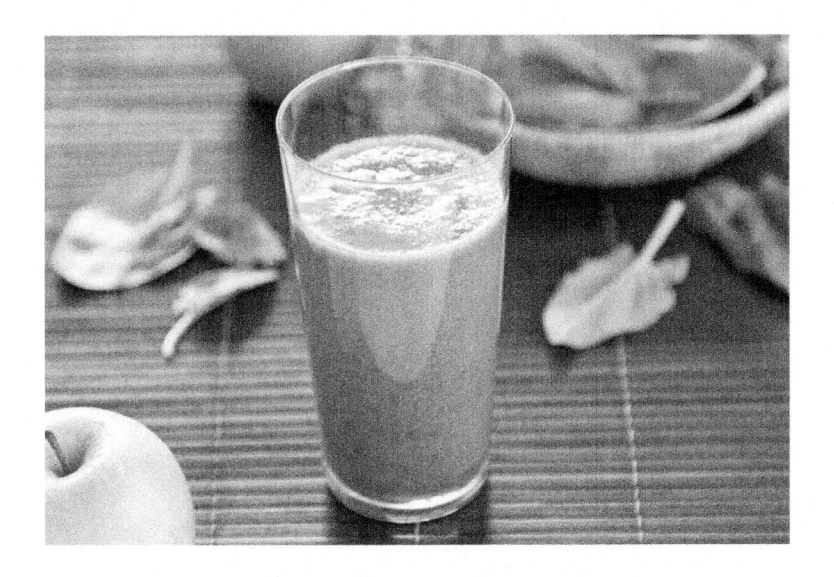

This is a very popular green detox juice. It balances veggies and fruits together so well. It's the perfect blend to use to detox your body following parties or holiday celebrations. Apples are packed with good nutrition, and they are an excellent source of vitamin C, and polyphenols, which give you a number of health benefits.

Makes 2 Servings

Prep Time: 7-10 minutes

Ingredients:

- 3 celery stalks, without leaves
- 2 halved apples, green
- 8 kale leaves
- 1 cucumber, no skin
- 1 pc. of ginger, fresh
- 1/2 peeled lemon
- Optional: mint sprig

Instructions:

1. Wash the vegetables and fruits thoroughly.

2. Cut or chop ingredients as needed. Remove peels.

3. Place ingredients in your juicer.

4. Process into healthy detox juice.

20 – Apple Cucumber Detox Juice

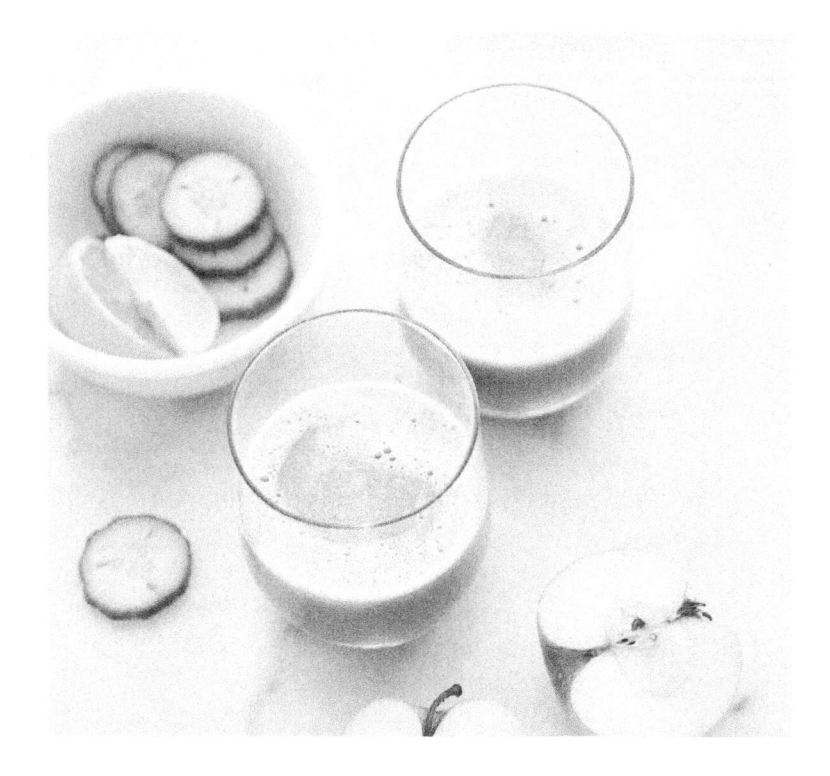

This recipe is another juice that is both delicious and easy to make. It has great detoxifying properties and it's also alkalizing and hydrating. The delicious taste will encourage you and your family to drink more of the juice, gaining its many benefits.

Makes 2 Servings

Prep Time: 10 minutes

Ingredients:

- 1 cup of parsley
- 1 cucumber
- 2 apples, green
- 1 cup of spinach leaves

Instructions:

1. Clean fruits and vegetables well.

2. Cut or chop ingredients as desired and remove rinds and peels.

3. Place ingredients in your juicer.

4. Process into detox juice.

21 – Turmeric and Carrot Detox Juice

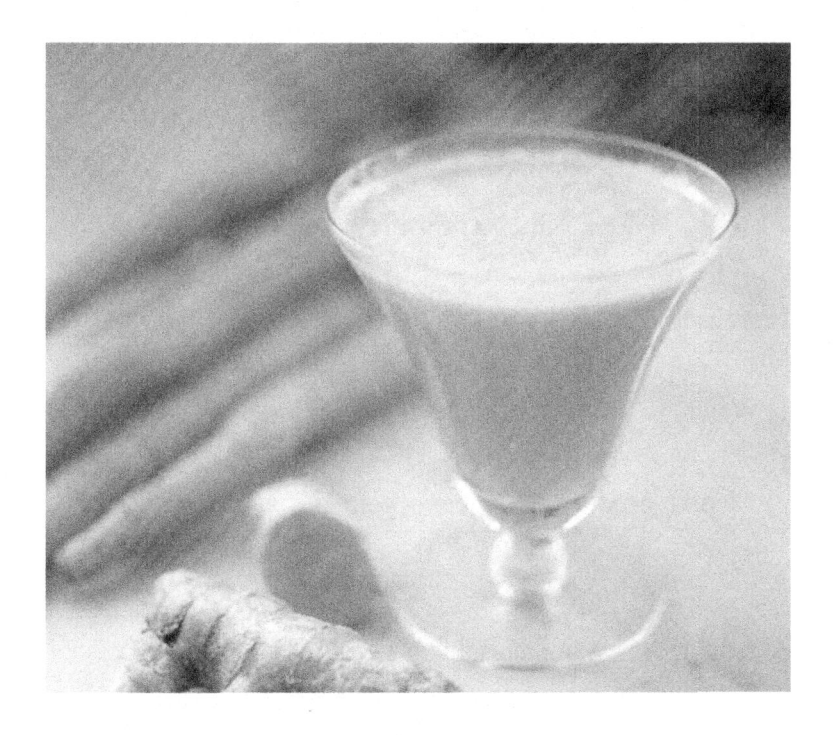

Not only is this a great way to remove toxins from your body, but it also helps you to maintain good eyesight with its healthy carrots.

Makes 4 Servings

Prep Time: 10-12 minutes

Ingredients:

- 2 or 3 oranges, navel
- 8 carrots, large
- 1 or 2-inch piece of ginger, fresh
- Optional: 1-inch of turmeric

Instructions:

1. Wash the produce to remove pesticides, etc.

2. Prepare produce for juicer – get rid of skins and rind and chop, if desired.

3. Add the ingredients to juicer.

4. Process produce into detox juice.

5. Serve chilled, if desired.

22 – Anti-Inflammatory Detox Juice Blend

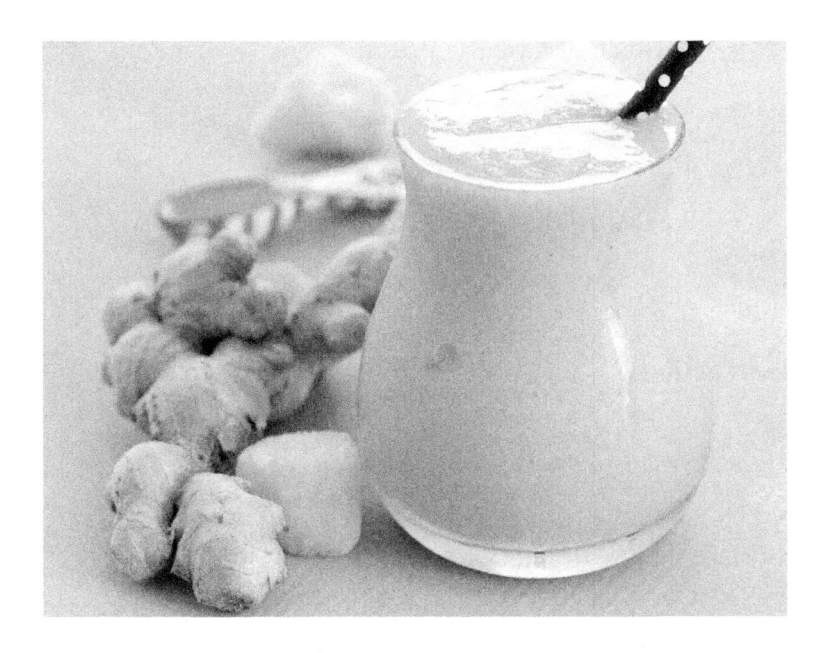

This energizing, anti-inflammatory juice is so helpful for your energy level and digestive tract. Try this juice in the mornings instead of your typical orange juice. You'll be glad you chose this nutrient packed drink.

Makes 2 Servings

Prep Time: 8-10 minutes

Ingredients:

- 4 carrots, medium
- 3/4-inch of turmeric, fresh
- 1 orange, navel
- 1/3-inch of ginger, fresh
- 3 celery stalks
- 1/2 lemon, rind removed

Instructions:

1. Wash the fruits and vegetables well.

2. Place them into juicer.

3. Process thoroughly.

4. Serve chilled.

23 – Orange and Ginger Detox Juice

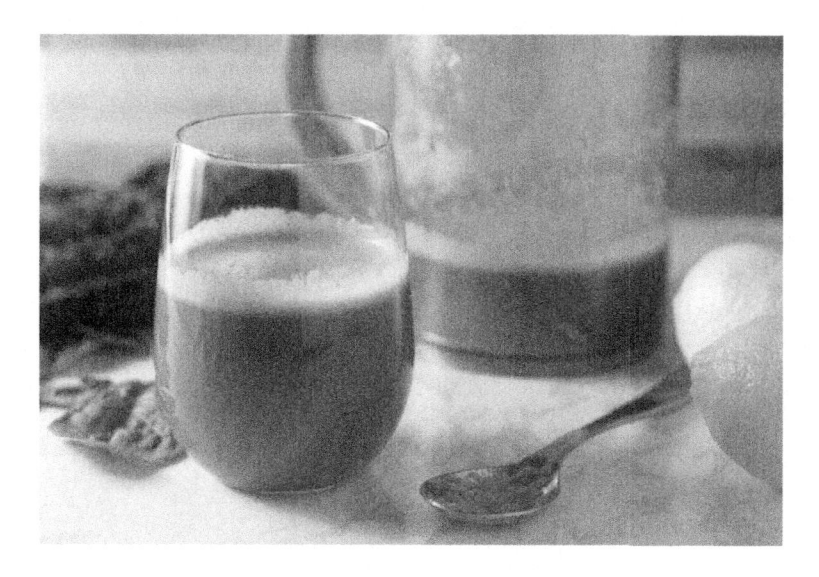

This is one of the tastiest detox juices you'll ever make. If you want a healthy drink that can also be used for weight loss, this is a great choice. This recipe is especially tasty in the summer, when the weather is warm, since it is also refreshing.

Makes 1 Serving

Prep Time: 6-8 minutes

Ingredients:

- 2 quartered beets, red
- 1 quartered apple, green
- 1 orange – remove the rind
- 3 carrots, large
- 1 handful of spinach leaves
- 1-inch piece ginger, fresh

Instructions:

1. Clean the fruits and veggies well.

2. Chop if desired before using juicer.

3. Add all ingredients to your juicer.

4. Process into detox juice.

5. Chill and serve.

24 – Pear and Kale Detox Juice

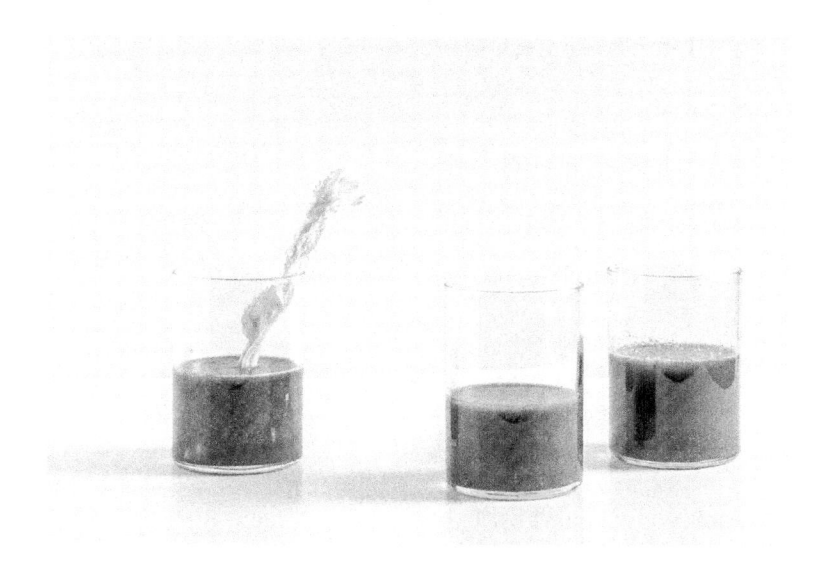

Sometimes, if you've done juicing before, your body will crave juices. This may seem rather unlikely unless you've tried a tasty detox juice like this one. Green juices CAN be refreshing and fruity, and this one is an excellent example. You'll find it much easier to include fruits and veggies in your diet when you juice them.

Makes 2 Servings

Prep Time: 10 minutes

Ingredients:

- 1 cup of spinach leaves
- 2 kale stalks
- 1/2 lime, no rind
- 1 pear, no skin
- 1/2 cucumber, peeled
- 3 celery stalks

Instructions:

1. Wash veggies and fruits before you juice.

2. Cut the veggies and fruits into 2-inch pieces, so the juicer can work more effectively.

3. Place produce in machine. Turn it on and allow it to run till it has extracted all juice.

4. Enjoy when juicer is done or chill and drink later.

25 – Sweet Apple and Carrot Detox Juice

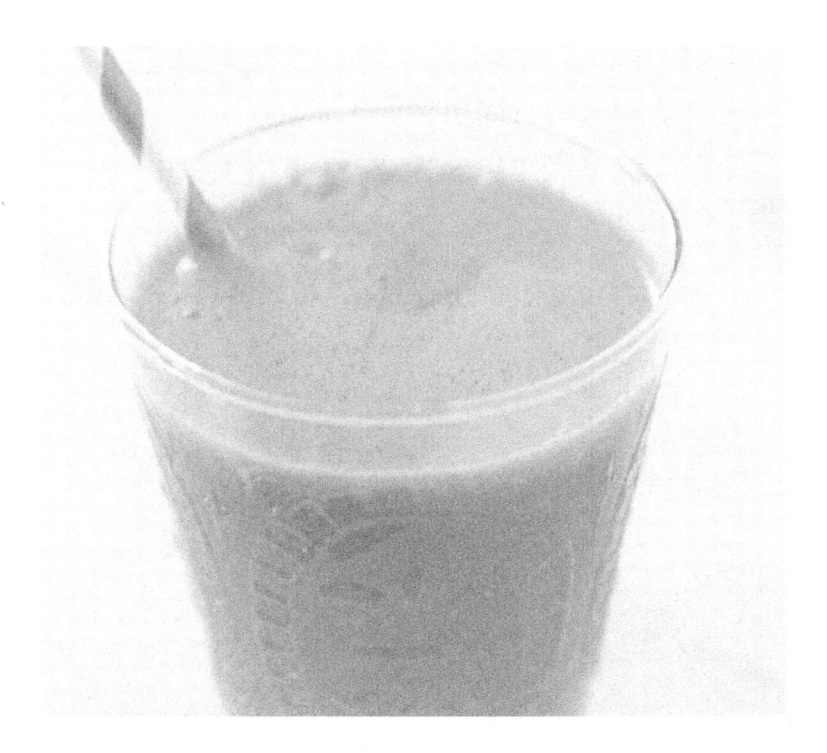

This recipe is a very healthy juice, and you can drink it nearly every morning without getting tired of it. It provides all the nutrients your body needs.

Makes 4 Servings

Prep Time: 10-12 minutes

Ingredients:

- 2 apples, medium, peeled
- 10 carrots, large
- Optional: 1/4 cup of parsley, fresh

Instructions:

1. Thoroughly clean the fruits and vegetables.

2. Chop produce into chunks if desired.

3. Place produce in your juicer.

4. Blend and make fresh detox juice.

26 – Healthy Beet Detox Juice

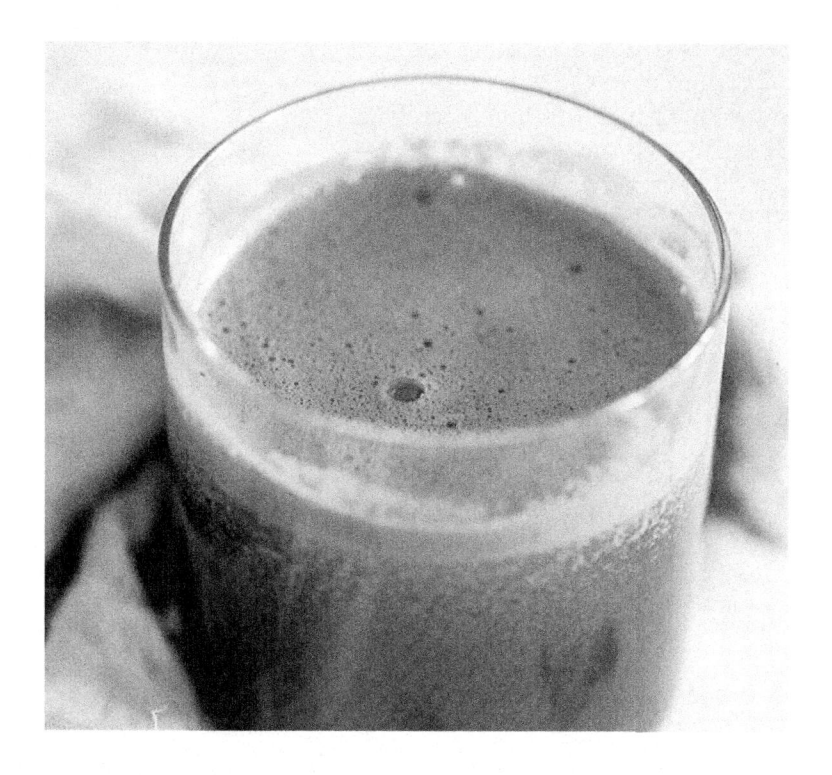

When you juice, it **Makes** it so much easier to make use of the nutrients in vegetables and fruits. This beet and ginger juice nourishes the body and aids it in getting rid of toxins. It's among the most popular of juices, too, because it is SO tasty.

Makes 2 Servings

Prep Time: 10 minutes

Ingredients:

- 3 beets, golden
- 1/2-inch of ginger, fresh
- 3 celery stalks
- 3 carrots, medium

Instructions:

1. Wash all produce well.

2. Cut or chop and remove skins and rind, if desired

3. Place produce in your juicer.

4. Process into healthy detox juice.

27 – Orange-Pineapple-Carrot Detox Juice

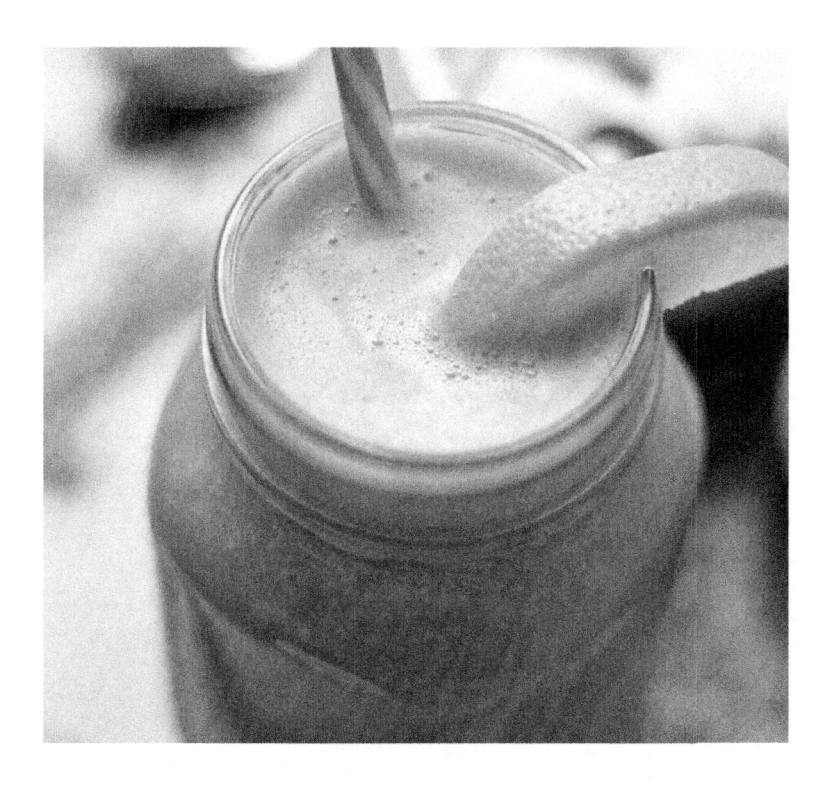

This is sometimes called a "dessert" juice, because it tastes so good. It tends to contain more sugar than green juices, since it uses more fruits. It's easy to make. It's much healthier for you than juices you buy at the store, since they have hidden ingredients and often add sugar, too. You'll love preparing juice yourself, so you know what's in it.

Makes 1 Serving

Prep Time: 6-8 minutes

Ingredients:

- 1 orange – remove the rind
- 9 medium carrots
- 1 slice of pineapple – remove skin
- 1 quartered apple, green
- 1" piece of turmeric root, fresh
- 1/2 lemon – remove rind

Instructions:

1. Clean veggies and fruits thoroughly.

2. Cut or chop if required for juicer.

3. Place all ingredients in your juicer.

4. Process into detox juice.

5. Serve chilled, if desired.

28 – Zingy Ginger Detox Juice

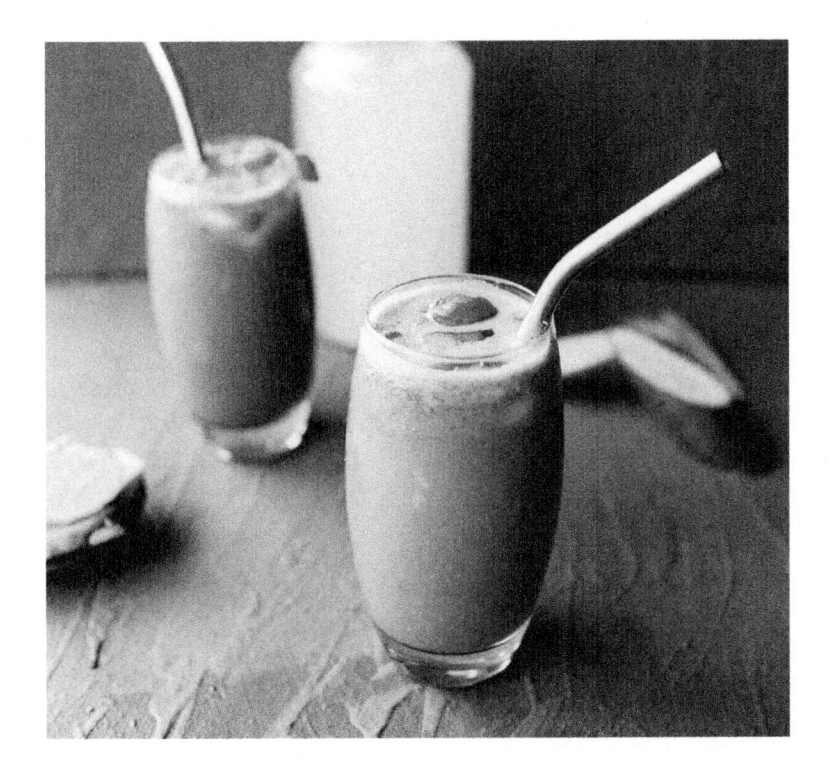

Ginger detox juice contains some super antibacterial properties. Ginger in its fresh form has long been known to be an effective anti-inflammatory. Ginger juice is also quite healthy for strong and long hair growth.

Makes 2 Servings

Prep Time: 10 minutes

Ingredients:

- 1/2 cucumber, skin removed
- 2 celery stalks
- 1/2 cup of parsley, flat leaf
- 1/2-inch piece of ginger, fresh
- 1 apple, green
- 1/2 lemon, no rind
- 2 cups of spinach leaves

Instructions:

1. Wash off the produce to eliminate traces of pesticides, etc.

2. Chop or chunk ingredients if desired, for your type of juicer.

3. Place produce into your juicer.

4. Blend and process into healthy juice.

5. Serve chilled, if desired.

29 – Almond Strawberry Detox Juice

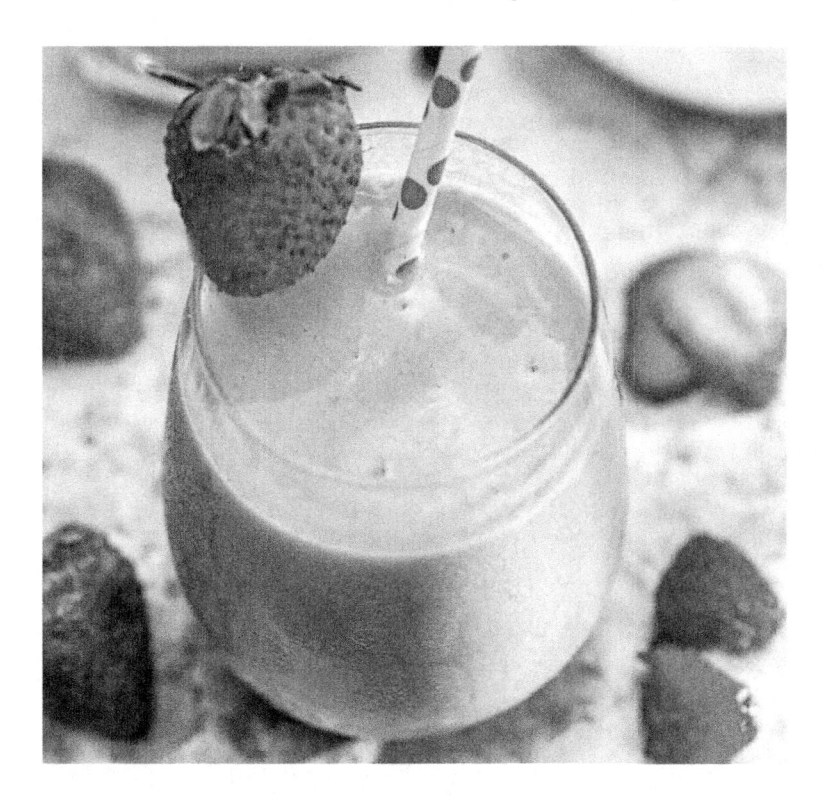

This is a newer spin on a long-time favorite detox recipe. It's a delicious and healthy alternative to straight juices or straight dairy drinks. It's refreshing and cool, and a great way for you to begin your day.

Makes 1 Serving

Prep Time: 6-8 minutes

Ingredients:

- 2 cups of water, filtered
- 1/2 cup of almonds, whole
- 1/2 tsp. of cinnamon, ground
- 1/2 tbsp. of agave nectar, pure
- 2 strawberries – remove the tops
- 1/2 a vanilla bean – remove seeds

Instructions:

1. Wash veggies and fruits before you juice.

2. Cut the veggies and fruits into 2-inch pieces, so the juicer can work more effectively.

3. Place produce in machine. Turn it on and allow it to run till it has extracted all juice.

4. Enjoy when juicer is done or chill and drink later.

30 – Tropical Mint Detox Juice

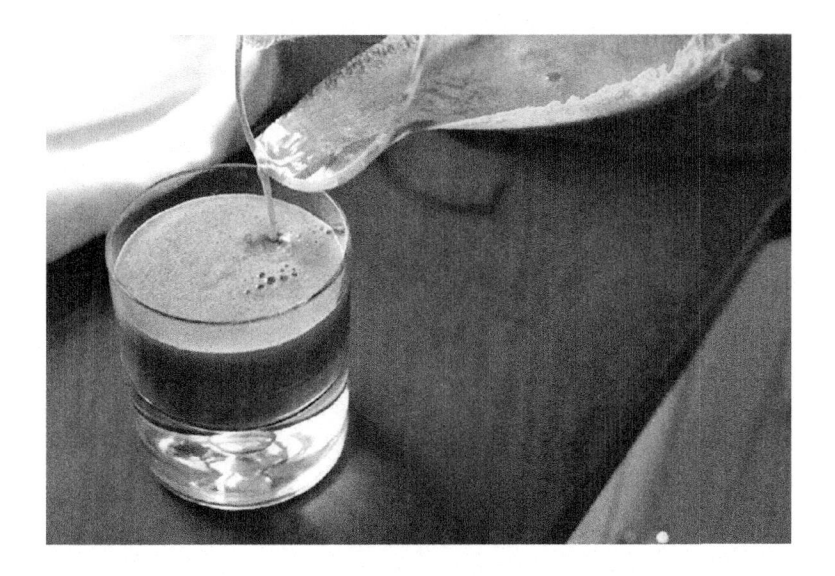

You can cool off anytime you like with a mint detox juice. Most juices are at least somewhat healthy for you, but this one adds some extra benefits, in addition to cleansing your body of toxins and assisting in weight loss. It can be helpful in improving your mood, too.

Makes 2 Servings

Prep Time: 10 minutes

Ingredients:

- 1/2 cucumber, no rind
- 2 celery stalks
- 3 cups of mint leaves, fresh
- 2 cups of spinach leaves
- 1/2 lemon, rind removed
- 1 cup of pineapple, chunked

Instructions:

1. Clean the produce well.

2. Chop or slice, if desired, for juicing.

3. Place the produce in your juicer.

4. Blend till consistency is smooth.

5. Serve chilled, if desired.

31 – Fruit-Free Detox Juice

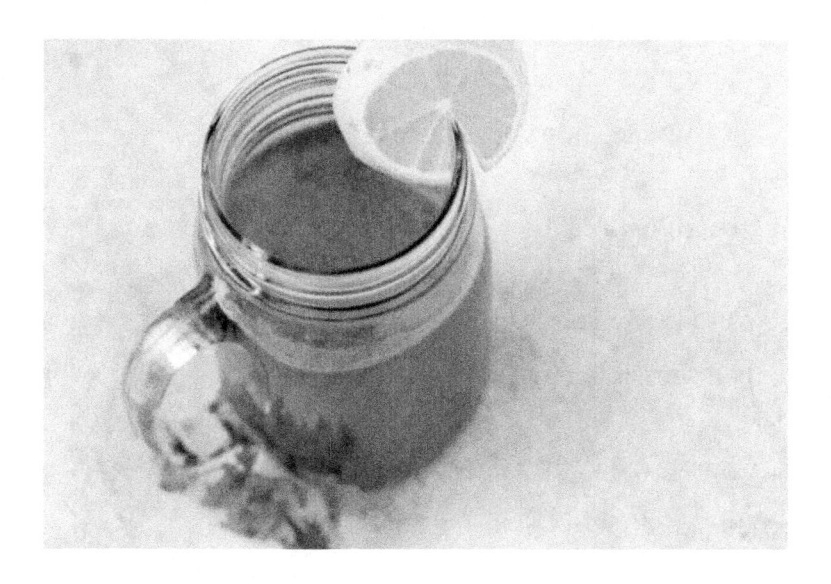

The detox juice comes to life when vegetables are juiced without fruit. This eliminates the calories found in even natural sugars, so it's a very healthy way to get the nutrients you need without the sugar.

Makes 2 Servings

Prep Time: 10-15 minutes

Ingredients:

- 1 bunch of carrots – removed tops
- 8 stalks of celery

- 1 bell pepper, red
- 1 x 1" knob ginger, fresh
- 1 lime – remove skin
- 1 bunch of parsley, flat-leaf

Instructions:

1. Wash the veggies well, to get rid of any residual pesticides and dirt possibly on them.

2. Chop or slice the vegetables if desired, or if your juice requires it. Remove skin and peels if desired

3. Place all produce in your juicer.

4. Process to make detox juice.

5. You can drink right away or put it in the fridge and drink it chilled.

32 – Super Natural Detox Juice

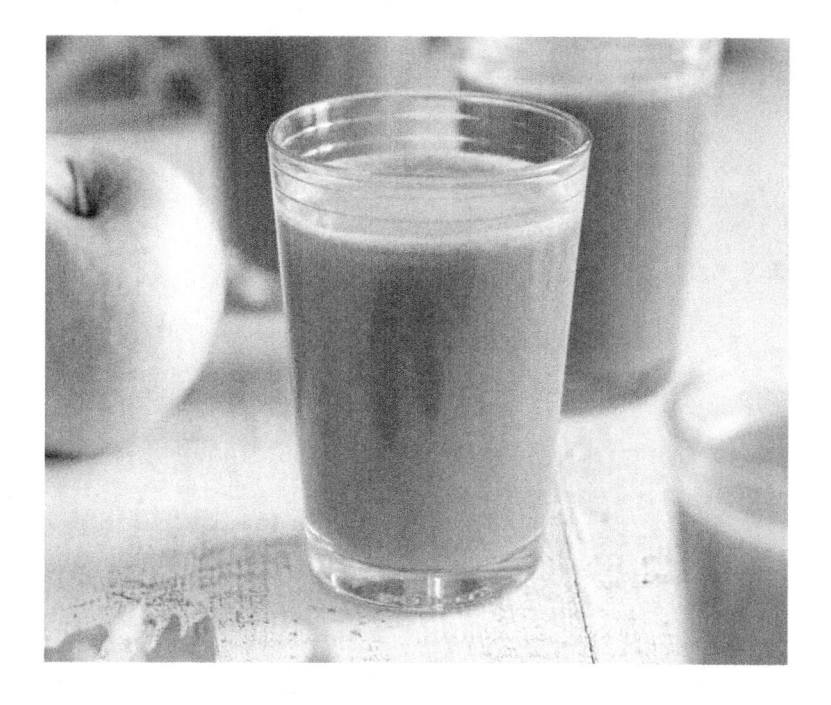

This isn't "supernatural", but it IS super detox juice that is, of course, all natural. The proteins are helpful in promoting your body's innate abilities of detoxification. This detox juice is beautiful to look at, but don't stop there. It offers loads of nutrients that help your body cleanse itself of toxins.

Makes 1 Serving

Prep Time: 10 minutes

Ingredients:

- 1 or 2 apples, green
- 3 or 4 leaves of kale
- 1 cucumber, chopped if desired
- 1 broccoli head
- A handful of flat-leaf parsley
- 1" piece pepper, jalapeno
- 1" piece ginger, fresh
- Optional for garnishing: turmeric, ground

Instructions:

1. Wash the produce well. You want to remove any chemicals or dirt, so they don't end up in your juice.

2. Remove apple core and broccoli stems.

3. Chunk or cut as desired, if your juicer requires smaller pieces, not whole produce.

4. Add ingredients to the juicer.

5. Process to make your detox juice. Garnish if desired with the ground turmeric and serve.

33 – Healthy Green Detox Juice

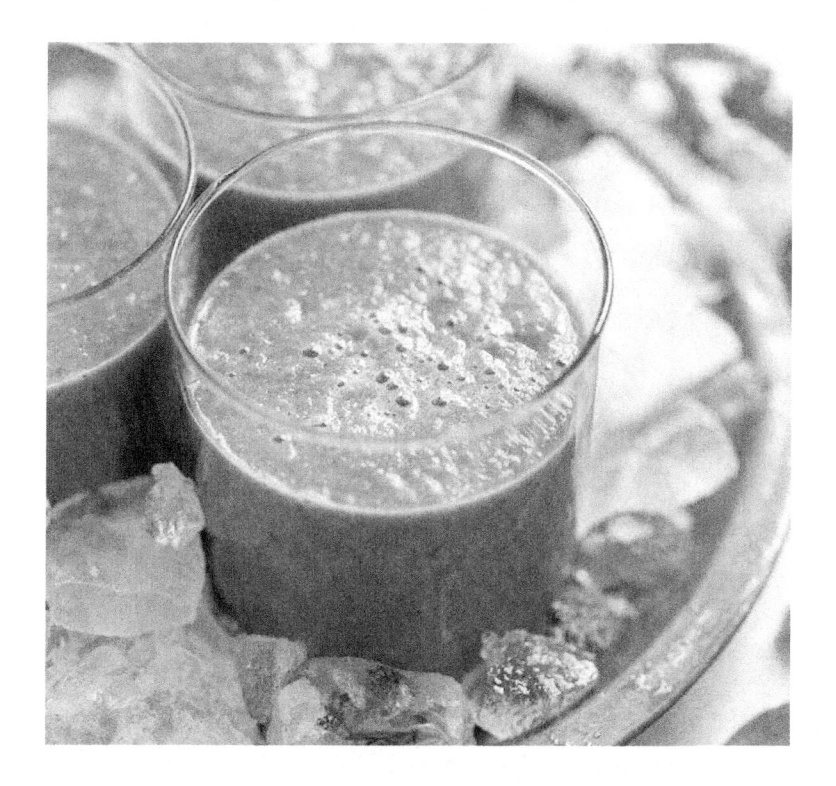

This is a wonderful and healthy juice to use for detoxing after you've had too much of the good things at parties or holiday meals. It tastes best if you buy organic celery, but you can make it with standard store-bought if you like. You can adjust the vegetable and fruit amounts depending on how sweet you like your juice. Adding apples will make your juice sweeter.

Makes 2 Servings

Prep Time: 10-12 minutes

Ingredients:

- 4 celery stalks, no leaves
- 2 halved apples, green
- 6 kale leaves
- 1 cucumber
- 1 x 1" piece of ginger, fresh
- 1/2 of 1 lemon, peel removed

Instructions:

1. Clean your produce well, so no dirt or residual chemicals can taint your juice.

2. Chop or cut veggies and fruits if your juicer won't take full produce. Remove the skin and peels, if desired.

3. Place ingredients in your juicer.

4. Process into detox juice.

34 – Cucumber Carrot Detox Juice

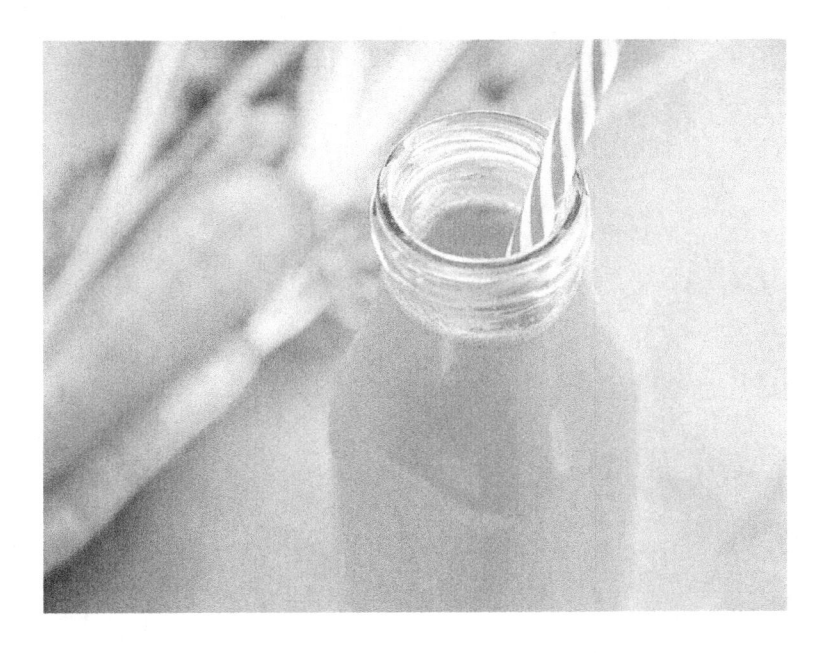

Today is the best day to adopt the healthy habit of juicing, of starting your day with tasty juice instead of a doughnut and coffee. This green juice will give you more energy as it detoxifies your body. It's the perfect choice if you haven't yet tried leafy green juices, since the taste is not as strong. It's a bit sweet, from the carrots, and very hydrating, from the cucumber.

Makes 1-2 Servings

Cooking + Prep Time: 8-10 minutes

Ingredients:

- 1 cucumber
- 3 or 4 carrots, medium
- 1/2 of lemon, peel removed
- 1/2 beet, sweet
- 1" of ginger root, fresh

Instructions:

1. Wash the fruits and vegetables thoroughly, to make your juice its healthiest.

2. Cut the produce into chunks, if desired, or if your juicer can't handle whole fruits and vegetables. Remove skin and peels, if desired.

3. Place the ingredients in your juicer.

4. Process the mixture into detox juice.

35 – Great Greens Detox Juice

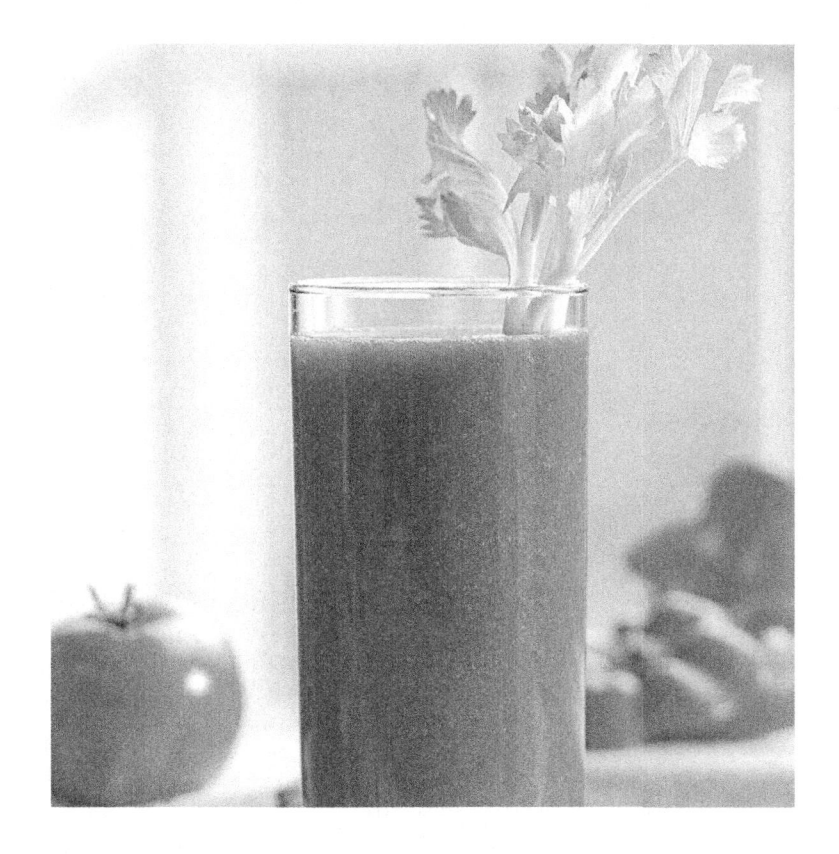

When you use fresh fruits and vegetables for juicing, the taste changes depending on whether the produce is in season or not, the ripeness and whether you purchase organic produce or not. This is a great juice to start with, and you can add in new ingredients, if you like, while still enjoying its wonderful taste.

Makes 1 Serving

Prep Time: 5-10 minutes

Ingredients:

- 1 asparagus spear
- 1 cucumber, rind removed
- 1 tomato, ripe
- 1/2 lemon, peel removed

Instructions:

1. Wash your produce well.

2. Chop or chunk-cut the fruits and vegetables if your juicer manufacturer recommends using pieces smaller than whole pieces of produce.

3. Remove peels or skins, as desired.

4. Place produce in your juicer.

5. Process the ingredients into detox juice. You can drink promptly or place it in the fridge and enjoy it chilled.

36 – Cabbage Carrot Detox Juice

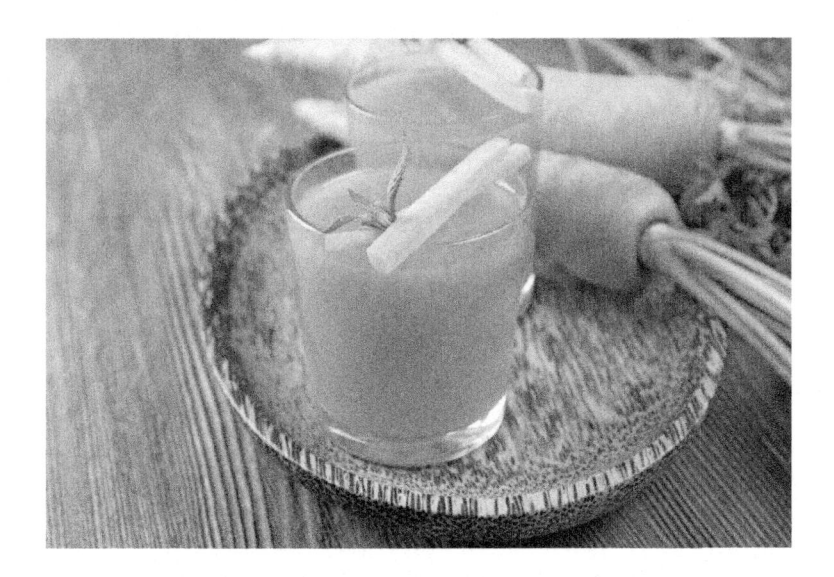

Cabbage is rarely used in juicing, but it has many positive attributes. It's often used in coleslaw recipes and in soups, and that helps to cleanse the body. But you can add wedges of it to any detox juice flavor. It adds nutrients to the recipe.

Makes 2 Servings

Cooking + Prep Time: 10-12 minutes

Ingredients:

- 3 peeled carrots, medium
- 1/4 head of cabbage, green

- 4 stalks of celery

Instructions:

1. Wash veggies and fruits before you juice.

2. Cut the veggies and fruits into 1 or 2-inch pieces, so the juicer can work more effectively.

3. Place produce in machine. Turn it on and allow it to run till it has extracted all juice.

4. Enjoy when juicer is done or chill and drink later.

37 – Tropical Pineapple Detox Juice

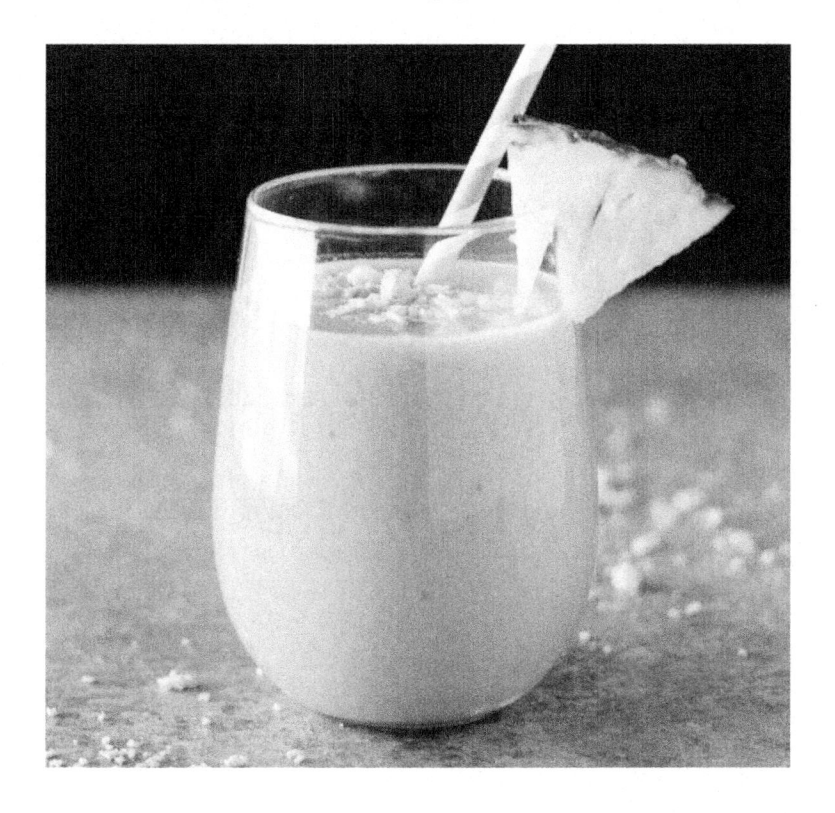

Are you tired of drinking detox juices that taste like all vegetables? If you want a sweet tasting juice, try the tropical flavors of this recipe!

Makes 1 Serving

Prep Time: 5-7 minutes

Ingredients:

- 2 carrots, large
- 1 quartered apple, large
- 2 pieces of ginger, fresh
- 1/4 pineapple, chunked

Instructions:

1. Wash veggies and fruits before you juice.

2. Cut the veggies and fruits as desired and remove skins and rinds if desired.

3. Place produce in machine and process.

4. Enjoy when juicer is done or chill and drink later.

38 – Healthy Skin Detox Juice

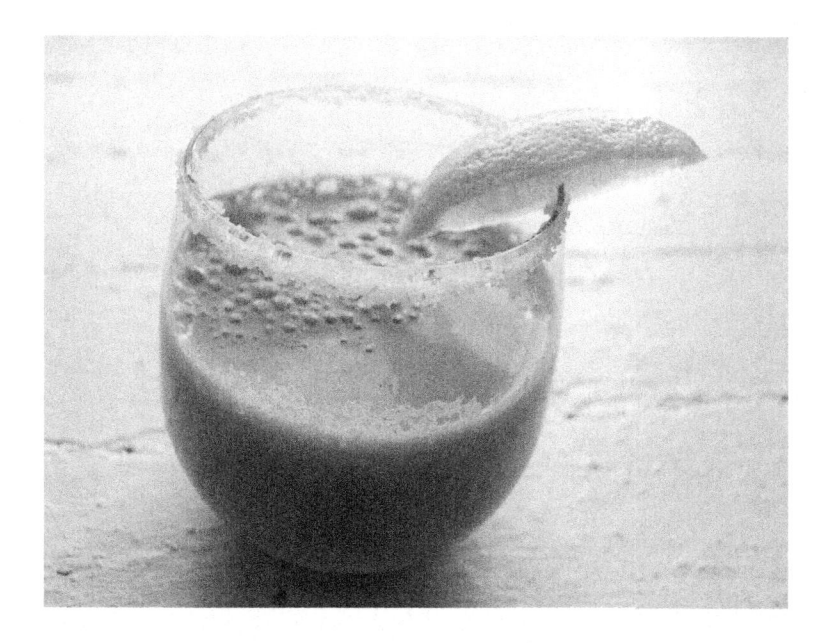

Bell peppers and cucumbers are excellent silicon sources. Silicon is recommended by dermatologists to strengthen your nails, skin and hair. Drinking silicon-enhanced detox juice helps you reduce wrinkles and other aging signs.

Makes 2 Servings

Prep Time: 10 minutes

Ingredients:

- 1 parsnip
- 1/4 pepper, green
- 1 cucumber
- 1/2 lemon, peeled
- 2 or 3 carrots, medium

Instructions:

1. Make sure produce is clean.

2. Slice or cube if needed for juicer. Remove peels and skins, if desired.

3. Place ingredients in juicer.

4. Use juicer to process the ingredients into detox juice.

39 – Energy Boost Detox Juice

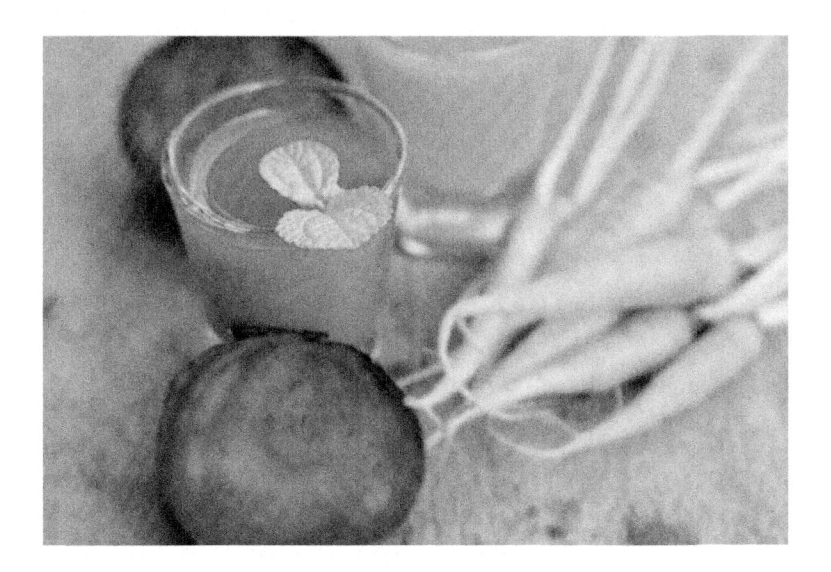

Here is a detox juice that cleanses the body as it gives you an energy boost. Enjoy one when you get up some mornings, to realize the complete effects.

Makes 1-2 Servings

Prep Time: 8-10 minutes

Ingredients:

- 2 beets, sweet
- 2 apples, green
- 2 carrots, medium

- 2 lemons, peeled

Instructions:

1. Wash vegetables and fruit before you juice.

2. Cut the produce into pieces of 2" or less so juice can be more thoroughly extracted.

3. Place vegetables and fruit into juicer. Turn it on and allow it to run uninterrupted till it extracts all the juice.

4. Enjoy juice as is or chill it first.

40 – Full Body Health Detox Juice

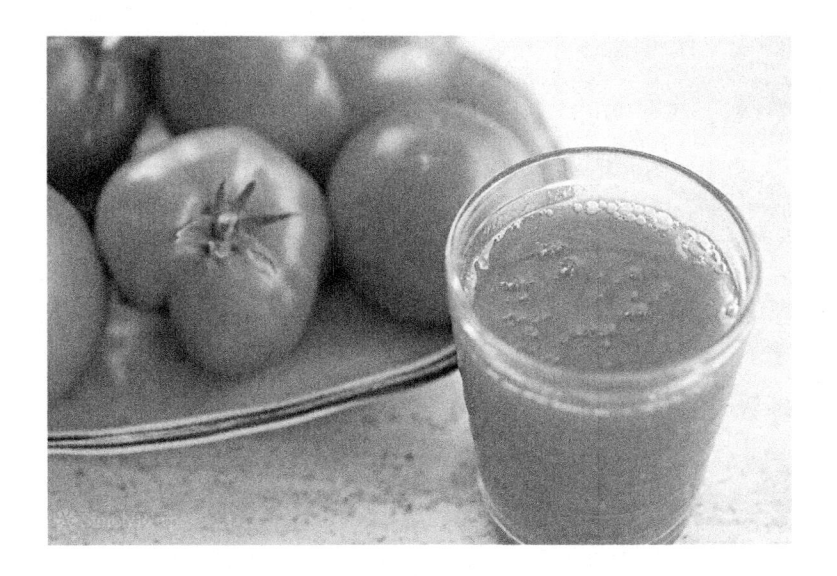

This juice is rich in chlorophyll, but that's far from being the only benefit. It's SO healthy and it tastes great, too. Asparagus contains a carb that isn't broken down in your intestine or stomach. Once it gets into the large intestine, it provides food for good bacteria. This lowers your chances of developing allergies. Asparagus even helps to reduce inflammation and lower blood sugar.

Makes 1 Serving

Prep Time: 5-7 minutes

Ingredients:

- 1/2 lemon, rind removed
- 1 cucumber
- 1 asparagus spear
- 1 tomato, ripe

Instructions:

1. Wash the ingredients thoroughly. Remove dirt and waxy areas.

2. Cut produce into chunks if that **Makes** it easier for your juicer to work. Remove peels and rind, as desired.

3. Place all the produce into the juicer.

4. Process into detox juice.

41 – Chia Berry Detox Juice

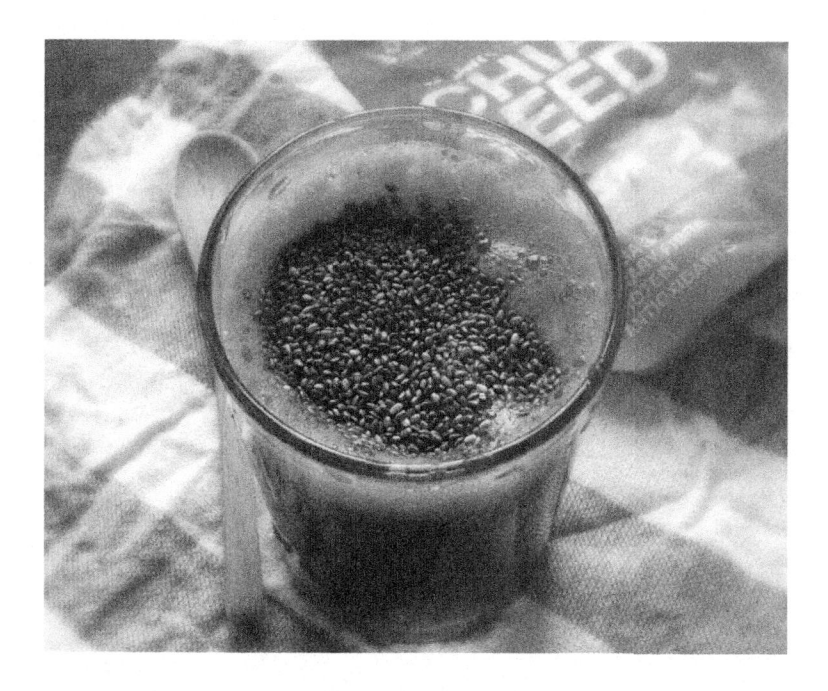

The chia seeds add fun to this tangy drink. You'll get more resveratrol than you can with red wine in this juice! It is rich in antioxidants and it works well to maintain healthy cholesterol and blood glucose levels. It's filled with manganese, folic acid, vitamins K and C and dietary fiber.

Makes 2 Servings

Prep Time: 8-10 minutes

Ingredients:

- 1 cup of de-stemmed kale leaves
- 1 quartered apple, large
- 1 cup of mixed berries, like blueberries, blackberries, raspberries or strawberries
- 5 large leaves of basil
- 2 tbsp. of chia seeds
- 1/2 cup of juice, pomegranate

Instructions:

1. Clean any unpeeled fruits and veggies well.

2. Cut produce into 2-inch pieces if your juicer instructions recommend it.

3. Place produce into the juicer.

4. Allow the juicer to continually run till all juice has been extracted.

5. You can drink juice when done, or chill and drink it later.

42 – Liver Cleanse Detox Juice

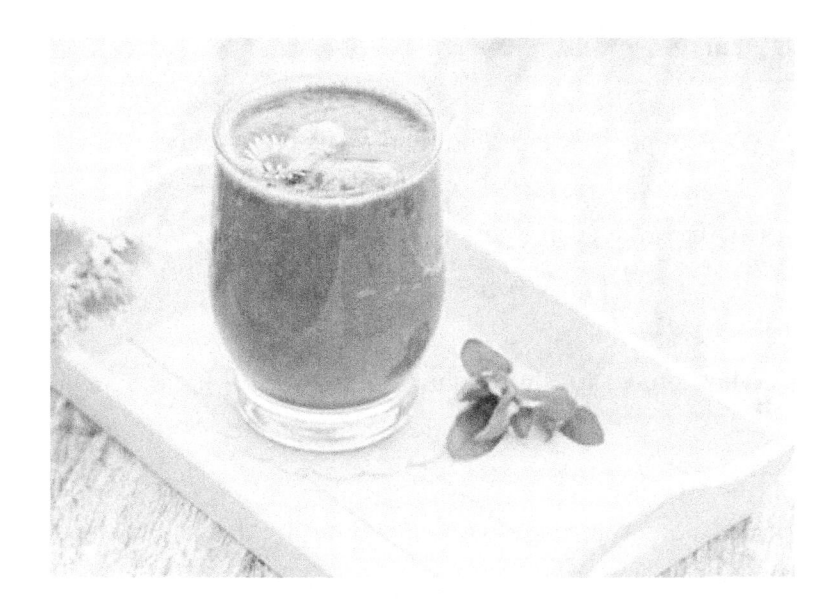

For many years, dandelion juice has been used for liver cleansing. You can add tincture of dandelion to any detox juice, if the greens are unavailable for you locally.

Makes 1 Serving

Prep Time: 5-10 minutes

Ingredients:

- 3 or 4 carrots
- 1 handful dandelion greens
- 1/2 peeled lemon

- 1/2 cucumber

Instructions:

1. Wash unpeeled vegetables and fruits thoroughly.

2. Cut the produce into small sized pieces if that enables your juicer to extract juice better.

3. Allow juicer to run without stopping it till it extracts all juice.

4. Enjoy juice when done, or place in the fridge and drink chilled.

43 – Earthy Taste Detox Juice

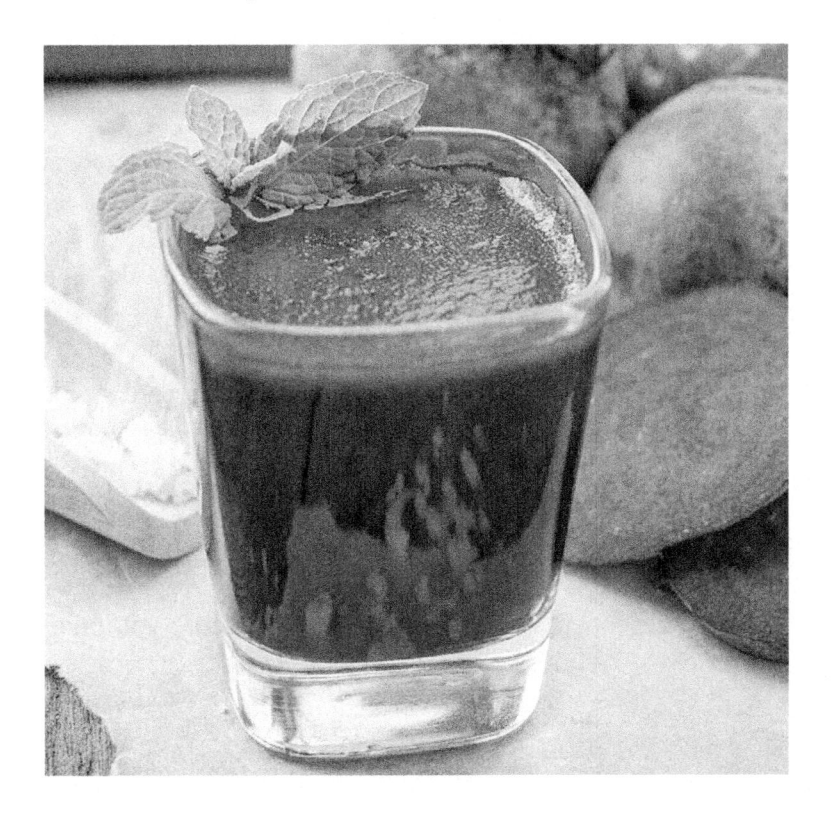

Earthy taste doesn't actually sound that appealing but give it a try – it is! It comes from the celery, beets and carrot. They help you to feel full. In addition, they are filled with vitamins, phytochemicals and antioxidants. This detox juice helps to lower blood pressure, even as it will stimulate digestion and flush out the kidneys.

Makes 1-2 Servings

Cooking + Prep Time: 5-7 minutes

Ingredients:

- 3 carrots, large
- 1 halved red beet, stems included
- 1 quartered apple, large
- 2 celery stalks, leaves included
- 2 leaves of mint
- 1 handful of parsley, flat leaf

Instructions:

1. Wash the unpeeled vegetables and fruit before you juice them.

2. Cut the produce into small pieces to get the juice more thoroughly.

3. Add produce to juicer and turn it on. Allow it to run uninterrupted till all juice is extracted.

4. Drink right away or chill and drink later.

44 – Sweet Veggie Detox Juice

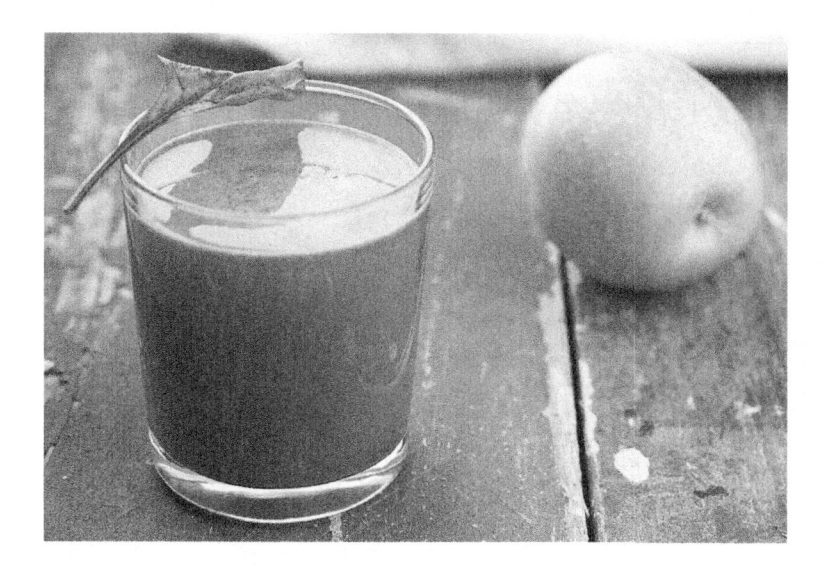

Adding lemon to your detox juice is like adding instant nutrition to juices. Many antioxidants can break down before reaching the bloodstream, but lemon helps them to be preserved and delivered.

Makes 1 Serving

Prep Time: 6-8 minutes

Ingredients:

- 4 leaves of romaine lettuce
- 3 leaves of kale with removed stems

- 2 apples, Fuji
- 1/2 lemon, peeled
- 1 small handful spinach leaves

Instructions:

1. Wash veggies and fruits before you juice.

2. Cut the veggies and fruits into 2-inch pieces, if desired.

3. Place produce in machine. Turn it on and allow it to run till it has extracted all juice.

4. Enjoy when juicer is done or chill and drink later.

45 – Healthy Ginger Lemon Juice

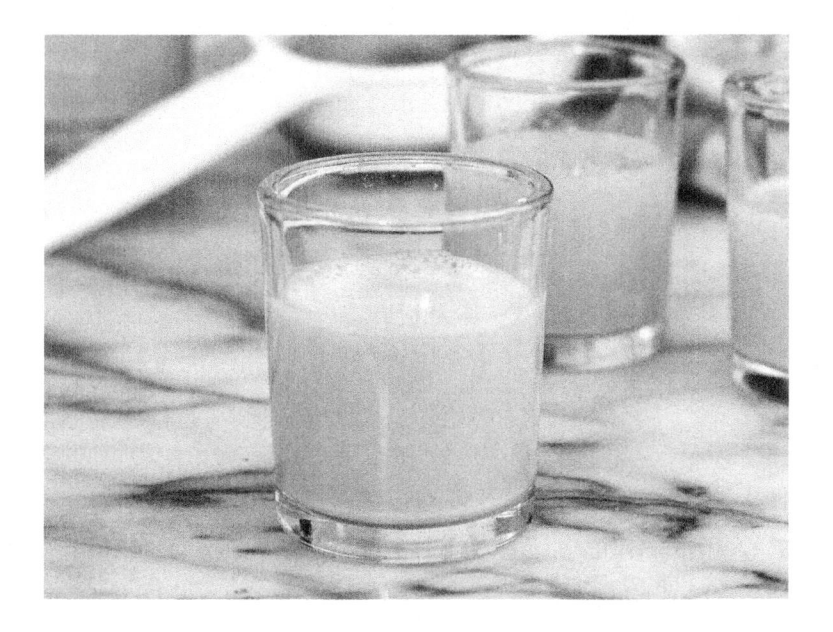

Lemons are helpful to your digestive tract. They also purify the blood, rid your body of dangerous toxins, fight free radicals and reduce joint inflammation. The vitamin C fights off the flu and colds. Ginger is soothing for the intestines, and it eases nausea. It also boosts your immunity to disease.

Makes 2 Servings

Prep Time: 6-8 minutes

Ingredients:

- 2 tbsp. of ginger root
- 2 lemons, juice only, with pulp
- 1 tbsp. of honey, pure
- 1 cups of water, hot

Instructions:

1. Wash vegetables and fruits well, to remove dirt and chemicals.

2. Cut the produce into 2" pieces, if your juicer instructions recommend it.

3. Place fruits and vegetables in juicer.

4. Turn machine on. Allow it to run till it has extracted all the juice.

46 – Grapefruit and Spinach Detox Juice

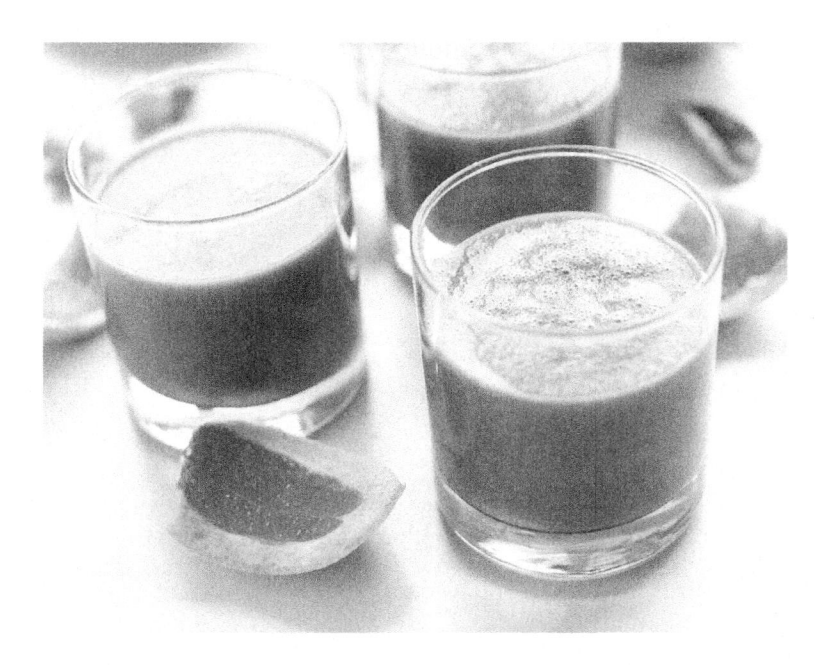

Sweetness and a bit of sourness combine in this detox juice. The grapefruit gives it a kick of sour. Blending and adding ice make it a cooler, more refreshing drink, and a thicker consistency.

Makes 1 Serving

Prep Time: 6-8 minutes

Ingredients:

- 1/2 ounce of mint, fresh
- 2 apples, Granny Smith
- 1 grapefruit, ruby red
- 8 ounces of spinach

Instructions:

1. Wash veggies and fruits well.

2. Cut produce into chunks if desired.

3. Place veggies and fruits in juice. Allow the machine to run till it has extracted all the juice.

4. Enjoy right away or pop in the fridge and drink chilled.

Conclusion

This detox juice cookbook has shown you…

… How to use different fresh fruits and vegetables to give your body the nutrition it needs each day.

How can you include juicing in your recipe repertoire?

It's easy! Follow one or two of the recipes in this book to start, and you'll see the instructions are very similar from one recipe to the next.

- Cleaning your produce is very important, before you toss it in the juicer. This step helps you get rid of pesticides and other materials that may be hiding on the skin, peel or rind of your fresh produce.
- Depending on the type of juicer you are using, you may need to chop the produce into chunks. Better or larger juicers will allow you to add your produce whole.
- Remove skin, rinds, seeds or peels if you like. This will give your juice a more consistent texture and make it easier to enjoy.

- Be sure to keep your juicer on long enough to make the result drinkable. It should be easy and rewarding to enjoy your detox juice.

You'll be so happy when you realize how easy it is to cleanse your body with detox juice. It gives your body the nutrients it needs the most, so you'll enjoy a healthier life. Have fun experimenting! Enjoy the results!

Printed in Great Britain
by Amazon